ENDURING ALZHEIMER'S

Practical Tips for Caring For Your Loved One and Yourself

MICHAEL BEHRMANN   DAN FOGARTY

BRUCE ALAN KEHR M.D.

 caringvillage

Contents

Disclaimer

Caring Village and the authors of this book (Michael Behrmann, Dan Fogarty, Bruce Kehr, and others) provides information (for example, health, legal, and financial) for informational purposes only, which should not be construed as advice. The information provided in this book, on our website ("Site"), or through links to other third-party sites, is not a substitute for obtaining proper medical, legal, financial or other professional care or services. We are not engaged in providing professional medical, legal or financial advice via this book, Site, or otherwise. You should not view the information provided in this book or on our Site as a substitute for medical, legal, or financial advice offered by a licensed professional or otherwise, and if necessary, you should seek the advice of a licensed medical, legal, or financial professional, as applicable. No action should be taken based upon any of the professional information contained in this book or our Site. You should seek independent professional advice from a person who is licensed and/or knowledgeable in the applicable area before acting upon any information contained within this book or Site. Caring Village and the authors of this book do not warrant the accuracy, completeness or currency of the information provided in this book or made available through our Site. Caring Village and the authors of this book do not accept any liability for any injury, loss or damage incurred by use of or reliance on the information contained within this book or our Site. Publication of the Content appearing in this book or on our Site does not necessarily constitute an endorsement of the views expressed therein and does not constitute a warranty or guarantee of any strategy, advice, recommendation, treatment, action, or medication. In addition, the materials in this book and on our Site may include sample or form agreements, letters or other documents, including financially or legally significant documents such as contracts and other items ("Forms"). Use of Forms does not constitute legal, accounting or other professional advice. Neither this book nor our Site should not be construed as providing specific instructions for individual patients, nor as a substitute for the diagnosis, treatment and advice of a medical or other professional. Any content contained in this book or on our Site should not be used to determine treatment for a specific medical condition. Health content does not cover all possible uses, precautions, side effects and interactions, and should not be construed as a representation or assurance that any drug or procedure is safe, appropriate or beneficial. Talk to a licensed doctor or pharmacist before using any prescription or over the counter drugs, including any herbal medicines or supplements. Only a licensed doctor or pharmacist can provide you with advice on what is safe and effective for you. You should also check the product information (including package inserts) regarding dosage, precautions, warnings, interactions, and contraindications before administering or using any device, drug, herb, vitamin, or supplement referenced or mentioned on this Site. For specific legal advice to rely on, you should seek advice from a lawyer, rather than this book or our Site. Any legal information provided in this book or our Site does not constitute legal advice. We make no claims, promises or guarantees about the accuracy, completeness, or adequacy of the legal information contained in this book or linked to our Site. Legal advice must be tailored to the specific circumstances of each matter, and laws frequently change. Nothing provided in this book or on our Site should be used as a substitute for the advice of competent legal counsel. This book and our Site do not make any recommendation or endorsement as to any financial investment, advisor or other service or product, or to any financial material submitted by third parties or linked to our website. In addition, our Site does not offer any advice regarding the nature, potential value or suitability of any particular investment, security or investment strategy. The financial information provided in this book and on our Site may not be suitable for your circumstance. If you have any doubts you should contact a qualified financial advisor. This book and our Site do not make recommendations for buying or selling any securities. It is up to users of this book and our Site to make their own financial decisions, and if necessary, to consult with a qualified financial advisor when evaluating the information in this book and on our Site.

ALL CONTENT THEREIN IS PROVIDED IN THIS BOOK "AS IS," "WITH ALL FAULTS" AND WITHOUT ANY WARRANTIES OF ANY KIND, EXPRESS OR IMPLIED. CARING VILLAGE AND THE AUTHORS OF THIS BOOK DISCLAIM ALL WARRANTIES WITH RESPECT TO THE SERVICES, EXPRESS OR IMPLIED, INCLUDING, BUT NOT LIMITED TO, WARRANTIES OF MERCHANTABILITY, FITNESS FOR A PARTICULAR PURPOSE, NON-INFRINGEMENT, TITLE, QUIET ENJOYMENT, MERCHANTABILITY OF COMPUTER PROGRAMS, DATA ACCURACY, SYSTEM INTEGRATION, AND

Foreword

Mike's Story

In the beginning of 2015, my mother-in-law was officially diagnosed with Alzheimer's Disease and joined the ranks of nearly 6 million Americans living with the disease. She was a tough and independent Scottish woman that was the rock of my wife's family. She was razor-sharp, quick-witted and took flak from no one. Her dynamic personality made it even harder for our family to comprehend how this horrible disease could affect her and filled us with fear as she started to lose her memory.

She rapidly transformed from the woman I had called "Mom" for 30 years to someone who couldn't remember her grand-children's names and threatened us with violence. Our entire family was instantly thrust into the role of caregiver(s). We had no prior experience, little to no understanding of the disease and no clue about the resources available to us. Our family struggled with constant miscommunication, legal challenges, and general chaos while caring for Mom. We learned very quickly how stressful caregiving truly can be.

While I was helping my family care for Mom, I realized I also had to care for my family. They were feeling the stress of caregiving, just like me. I had to be there for them with emotional support, guidance, and strength. I had to step up and support the family in ways I had never had to before. I became some sort of a "caregiver of caregivers."

It becomes easy to overextend yourself. The stress, the lack of sleep, the tension at work, or home all take a toll on you and your family. You start to see how it gets harder and harder to do the things you need to do to take care of yourself. You start to see how your family's health and well-being begin to deteriorate. Instead of a healthy dinner with the family you find yourself grabbing fast-food on the way to an appointment. Instead of getting a good night's sleep on your own bed, you find yourself curled up on a sofa. Instead of a jog around the neighborhood and a nice hot shower, you find yourself stressing out, going over paperwork again, and running out of steam.

The most applicable advice I have ever received about caregiving came from a flight attendant message to passengers, which we all have heard: "In the unlikely event of an emergency, oxygen masks will drop down from the overhead compartment. Make sure that your own oxygen mask is on first before helping your children." The most important thing you can do for your loved one is to take good care of yourself. It sounds backward, but it's true. Because if you're not taking care of yourself. How can you possibly provide care for someone else? Our hope in developing this book is to help you recapture some of your time, reassure you that it's okay to take time to take care for yourself, and most importantly spend time with the people you love. This is a time when families should be coming together, not drifting apart.

We are not here to tell you that there is a magic fix that will make everything better overnight, rather to give you a better understanding of the disease you and your family are facing, actionable plans and checklists to help you prepare for the unknown, and a comprehensive listing of resources available to you to help you on your journey.

~ Mike

Mike Behrmann is the CEO of Caring Village - a company devoted to helping families gain access to information and resources to care for those that they love.

How to Use this Book

We understand first-hand that the one thing you likely lack right now is time. Keeping that in mind, we developed this book so that it does not have to be read sequentially. Feel free to use the table of contents as your guide to focus on the items of need that are most important to you now. We have worked, and continue to work, over the last several years to compile resources from experts in numerous fields, families that have gone through what you are going through, and professional caregivers. We have also included information from our own personal caregiving experiences in an effort to create a guide to understanding and actionable steps. We are also very interested in suggestions for new topic areas or questions so if you find yourself curious about a topic that we don't cover, do not hesitate to contact us directly here.

What is Alzheimer's Disease and Dementia?

ONE

What is Alzheimer's?

According to the National Institute on Aging, Alzheimer's disease is "an irreversible, progressive brain disorder that slowly destroys memory and thinking skills and, eventually, the ability to carry out the simplest tasks. In most people with Alzheimer's, symptoms first appear in their mid-60s." Alzheimer's disease is the most common cause of dementia among older adults, and the risk of getting it increases with age.

The disease begins with an abnormal accumulation of proteins within the brain. These proteins are called beta-amyloid plaque and tau tangles and are the most common markers of Alzheimer's. The brain functions optimally by transmitting billions of neurons to distribute information to specific areas of the brain. Those messages are then communicated to the rest of the body. The proteins developing as a result of Alzheimer's prevent healthy neurons from working properly, and then they lose their ability to function and communicate with each other, and the neurons eventually die (source). The damage at first appears to take place in cells of the hippocampus, the part of the brain essential in forming memories.

These changes may take a decade or more to result in noticeable symptoms. Those diagnosed with Alzheimer's often display symptoms, including memory loss, problems with communication, loss of mobility, problems with incontinence, and other significant behavioral changes.

"I found for my dad, the pragmatic use of language - conversational give and take we use to connect with others - faded well before his desire to be connected and his rather prodigious vocabulary. Questions and scripted stories where what he had left to engage with. For him, it's the first time; for you, it's Groundhog Day."

It is important to remember that Alzheimer's disease destroys nerve connections in the brain, but the disease is not actually what kills. Complications of the decline in brain function are what led to death.

The common cause of death (of Alzheimer's) is a severe infection due to the impairment of the immune system. The most common infection is aspiration pneumonia – when food or liquid goes down the windpipe instead of the esophagus, causing damage or infection in the lungs that develops into pneumonia (source).

TWO

What are the Warning Signs of Alzheimer's?

The most common warning signs and symptoms for Alzheimer's to look for include:

- Losing things or misplacing items in odd places
- Rapid mood and/or personality changes
- Poor judgment and decision making
- Repeating questions over-and-over again
- Trouble completing normal, routine tasks
- Significant memory loss disrupting daily life
- Confusion with the time and location of where they are
- Problems with reading and writing
- Withdrawal from regular activities

Displaying one symptom is not an immediate cause for concern, but anything abnormal should be discussed and documented with a physician. Memory loss does not necessarily mean Alzheimer's, but pay attention to regular day-to-day activities, mood changes, and the other items listed above.

At this time, there is no known cure for the disease, but treatments are available to help manage the symptoms in some people. Alzheimer's is one of the most widely researched biomedical diseases and will continue to receive research funding until a cure is found.

THREE

What is Dementia?

Are you or someone you care about misplacing objects and unable to retrace the steps to find them? Is it difficult to make simple meals you've made hundreds of times before? Do friends or relatives complain that they've already answered the question you just asked? Are you becoming more forgetful, for example, repeatedly forgetting important appointments or other commitments you have made? This type of forgetfulness is oftentimes associated with Dementia; however, it could actually be a sign of:

- Normal Age-Related Memory Loss
- Dementia
- Mild Cognitive Impairment
- A result of Bipolar Disorder or Depression
- Delirium
- Side effects caused by medication
- Underlying medical conditions

Aging and the different types of memory loss or signs of dementia can be confusing. Don't let concerns about memory loss tangle your mind in your golden years.

Normal Age-Related Memory Loss

Just as we physically slow down through the years, so do our minds. As we age, our brains don't work as fast to learn new information or retrieve the old information we have stored in our memory banks. General forgetfulness is common in older adults. However, if you give yourself a few moments, the information should eventually come to mind. You may start to describe a book you are reading and then suddenly forget the title. You may walk outside to your car only to forget where you were headed. These age-related mishaps in memory can be frustrating but should not be a cause for alarm.

Dementia

Dementia is not a specific disease but rather a group of symptoms. These symptoms generally include memory loss, personality changes, and impaired reasoning. One in three people over 65 will develop dementia. Dementia usually affects those over the age of 60, but it is not a normal part of aging.

Dementia is caused when the brain is damaged by diseases, such as Alzheimer's disease or a series of small strokes. It can be associated with other conditions such as Parkinson's disease or Down's Syndrome. Risk factors, besides age, include infectious diseases (for example, HIV and syphilis), vascular (blood vessel) disease, depression, and chronic drug or alcohol abuse.

Dementia is often progressive, which means the symptoms will gradually get worse. However, some types of dementia – approximately 20% – are reversible. The most common types of reversible dementias are depression, the adverse effects of certain prescription or nonprescription drugs, drug or alcohol abuse, brain tumor, and metabolic and hormone conditions like hypothyroidism, and nutritional conditions like vitamin B-

12 deficiency. Depression is by far the most common of the potentially reversible conditions.

Mild Cognitive Impairment (MCI)

Mild Cognitive Impairment (MCI) is a brain impairment with a degree of severity that lies between normal memory lapses and dementia. It is usually an intermediate stage between the expected mental decline of normal aging and the more-serious decline of dementia. Not only memory is affected though, it can also involve problems with language, thinking, and judgment. The diagnosis of MCI relies on the fact that the individual is still able to perform all of their usual daily activities.

Cognitive Impairment in Bipolar Disorder and Depression

Memory loss can also co-occur with major mood disorders. For instance, in bipolar patients who experience depression and mania, research has shown that there are lapses in recalling a specific event in the past – such as a birthday celebration or concert. This deficit applies to the person's unique experience of the event. In addition, working memory – a function of the brain that processes and manipulates short-term memories – can also be impaired. In contrast, depressed patients, with no manic episodes, may experience memory loss in recalling specific events in the past. Depression can predispose to signs of memory loss, making it hard for you to concentrate, stay organized, remember, and get things done.

Delirium vs. Dementia

According to the Mayo Clinic, "delirium is a serious disturbance in mental abilities that results in confused thinking and reduced awareness of your environment." Delirium is typically caused by severe physical illness or toxic drugs and has a rapid onset. Delirium is often reversible while dementia typically has a slower onset, and is generally irreversible. Because symptoms of delirium and dementia can be similar, a careful history of symptom onset and progression from a family member or caregiver may be important for a doctor to make an accurate diagnosis.

What to Do Next

The good news is that, with proper diagnosis and treatment, in many instances, these worrisome symptoms can be reversed, or at least prevented from rapidly progressing. Seek help to differentiate between the various stages and types of memory loss to see if you need to take action. Feel free to reach out to Potomac Psychiatry for more information.

[i] Cognitive Impairments in Major Depression and Bipolar Disorders. Philip D. Harvey, Psychiatry 2007 Jan; 4(1): 12–14. Published online 2007 Jan. PMCID: PMC2922383. https://www.ncbi.nlm.nih.gov/pmc/articles/PMC2922383/

FOUR

Signs of Dementia

"I can't recollect certain events, places, and names. I routinely forget where I put things. And recently, I forgot the name of our pet. I used to call its name multiple times throughout the day. This behavior really has me worried. How can I forget a name I use every day?"

Each person's experience with dementia can be unique. It can vary from having only one or two symptoms to all of the following symptoms. The symptoms can also vary in severity. Sometimes symptoms are mild for a long time and only severe after a specific event, such as a stroke. The following are eight key symptoms of dementia that may cause concern.

1. Memory loss – this includes things such as forgetting the current president of the United States or the address where one has lived for some time.

2. Difficulty completing familiar tasks – for example, getting dressed in the morning or paying a bill.
3. Problems communicating – such as using the wrong word or forgetting simple words or being at a loss to express feelings and thoughts.
4. Disorientation – such as getting lost walking home from a store that is only a few blocks from one's house.
5. Problems with abstract thinking – such as managing finances (creating a budget or handling money transactions).
6. Misplacing things – forgetting where you left items and not being able to retrace your steps to eventually find them.
7. Mood changes – for example, swings in your mood from feeling very happy to very sad without an apparent reason.
8. Personality changes – becoming angry, suspicious, or fearful with loved ones or close friends. This may also include outbursts of aggression.

It's also worth mentioning that some conditions may cause people to be more likely to develop dementia. These include poor nutrition and chronic depression, genetics, and multiple concussions. In several studies of football players and professional boxers, repeated concussions and traumas to the head have shown an association with a greater risk for the development of dementia symptoms as they age. Dementia from concussions and traumatic brain injuries are irreversible.

FIVE

Types of Dementia

Now that you know the signs that are directly related to dementia, it's important to know some of the common types of dementia.

Alzheimer's Disease

There are many diseases and conditions that could cause or be associated with the symptoms of dementia, but Alzheimer's disease is the leading cause. Alzheimer's accounts for approximately 70% of all cases of dementia in the United States. According to the Alzheimer's Association, nearly 5.4 million Americans are currently living with the disease, and the biggest risk factor is advanced age (60 or older).

Dementia caused by Alzheimer's is progressive, which means the symptoms will gradually worsen over time. Alzheimer's develops slowly over a span of 20 or 30 years, and the diagnosis is often made when the disease process has been underway for many years. Genetic, environmental, and lifestyle factors may all play a role in the progression of brain cell damage and death over a period of decades.[i] It is eventually a fatal disease. In fact, Alzheimer's disease is the sixth leading cause of death in the U.S. for adults.

Familial Alzheimer's Disease

One rare form of Alzheimer's disease is known to be genetic. This is called Familial Alzheimer's disease (FAD). FAD accounts for between 2-3% of all cases of Alzheimer's and usually has an earlier onset with symptoms developing in their 30's or 40's. Genetic testing can determine if one has the gene for FAD.

Vascular Dementia

The second most common type of dementia is vascular dementia, which can occur after a series of small strokes. It is caused by brain damage from impaired blood flow to the brain. One can develop vascular dementia after a stroke blocks an artery in the brain, but strokes don't always cause vascular dementia. Vascular dementia can result from other conditions that damage blood vessels and reduce circulation to the brain, such as chronic high blood pressure, high cholesterol, and diabetes. Vascular dementia is generally irreversible, although lifestyle modifications and medication that normalize these three diseases can slow the progression.

Lewy Body Dementia

Dementia with Lewy bodies is a brain disorder linked to abnormal proteins in the brain. These deposits of proteins, called Lewy bodies, change the normal chemical make-up that allows your brain to function properly. The presence of Lewy bodies leads to problems with thinking, movement, behavior, and mood – all symptoms of dementia.

Other Faces of Dementia

Approximately 20% of the types of dementia are reversible and not progressive. Dementia symptoms that stem from nutritional deficiencies, such as a lack of B vitamins, are reversible, preventable, and generally mild. Not drinking enough liquids and not getting enough thiamin (vitamin B-1), which is common in people with alcoholism, and not getting enough vitamins B-6 and B-12 in your diet can all also cause dementia-like symptoms.

Chronic and severe depression can also cause dementia-like symptoms, which are also reversible. Symptoms that are common in depression and dementia include:

1. Loss of interest in activities and hobbies.
2. Social withdrawal
3. Trouble concentrating.
4. Impaired thinking
5. Memory problems
6. Sleeping too much or too little

A careful diagnostic process by a psychiatrist is necessary to determine if the symptoms the individual is experiencing are signs of depression, dementia, or both. This is why it's so important to seek treatment when feeling depressed or noticing the signs of dementia.

Unfortunately, most types of dementia, such as Alzheimer's, Vascular, and FAD, are irreversible, and there is no known cure. However, there is still much about the progression of dementia and the different diseases and conditions that cause it that are still unknown. Scientists and researchers have been ramping up their efforts to stem and cure diseases that cause dementia. In the meantime, there are some interventions that can slow the progression of dementia symptoms, and the symptoms may even be reversible. Recent research has pointed toward some promising nutritional and lifestyle interventions. There is hope.

SIX

Diagnosing Dementia

"My mother is 97 years old. I noticed that she was neglecting her chores, like cleaning her room or taking a shower as she used to do. She started hoarding and would get upset if I tried tidying up her closet. She can still hold a simple conversation, but her logic sometimes worries me, and I'm afraid to leave her home alone because she might hurt herself or leave the house and get lost. She refuses to go to be evaluated, and I don't know how to handle her dementia without getting her upset."

Diagnosing dementia and its subtype, or cause is like putting together the pieces of a difficult puzzle. Some of the pieces can go in multiple spots, and the pieces may all be similar in color or hue. Doctors can usually determine that a person has dementia with confidence. However, it is more difficult to pinpoint the exact type or cause of the dementia so that one would know if it is reversible or irreversible which, in turn, determines the treatment and care moving forward.

Scientific Definition of Dementia

Before we discuss the types of tests to determine the cause or type, let's discuss the criteria that doctors use to determine a diagnosis of dementia in the first place. Doctors turn to the DSM or Diagnostic Statistical Manual for the definition and criteria to use. The fifth edition of this manual, DSM-5, defines dementia as a "major neurocognitive disorder." To be considered a major neurocognitive disorder, there must be significant mental decline from previous mental performance on a variety of tests or scoring below what is considered "normal cognitive function" for the general population. What do we mean by significant mental decline when it comes to diagnosing dementia?

- The mental decline must cause problems for the individual or interfere with their ability to complete essential everyday tasks by themselves.
- The doctor must rule out delirium and other mental disorders such as depression.

A diagnosis of dementia requires "significant mental decline" in at least two core mental functions. The core mental functions are:

- Memory
- Language skills
- Ability to focus and pay attention
- Reasoning and problem-solving
- Visual perception

Core mental function abilities can be documented by the

physician using screening tests such as the Mini-Mental State Examination (MMSE) and the Montreal Cognitive Assessment (MoCA).

Tests to Define the Cause or Type of Dementia

As we discussed previously, dementia is not a disease itself but a cluster of symptoms. These symptoms of dementia can be caused by a wide variety of conditions. Some are physical, some are mental, and may even include lifestyle factors. It is vital that any patient who may be suffering from dementia receive a comprehensive workup. There are four main categories of testing used to help determine the cause or type of dementia. They are:

1. Mental and psychological
2. Physical and laboratory
3. Medical and lifestyle inventory
4. Brain imaging

Once the dementia diagnosis has been determined, it may be even more important to determine the cause or subtype because this will determine if it is reversible or irreversible and the steps moving forward for treatment and care.

Mental and Psychological Assessments

A psychologist or psychiatrist will examine a patient for any mental health conditions that could be causing the symptoms, which may include formal psychological testing. A mental health professional can determine whether chronic or severe depression is the main cause of the dementia. As previously mentioned, Depression is one of the most common causes of reversible dementia. Other mental health disorders, such as

Bipolar depression and schizophrenia, can hinder brain functioning as well.

Physical and Laboratory Testing

A person with suspected or confirmed dementia should have blood tests to check their overall level of physical health. Simple blood tests can sometimes detect problems that can affect brain function, such as vitamin B1, B6 or B12 deficiency. The thyroid should be tested for proper functioning as well. A physician should also consider testing the spinal fluid for infection, inflammation, or markers of some degenerative diseases. Nutritional deficiencies can be treated, and in many cases, reverse the dementia symptoms.

Medical and Lifestyle Inventory

Doctors will also review current prescription and over-the-counter medications to see if what is currently being prescribed could cause the symptoms of dementia. They will also ask about lifestyle factors that can cause dementia, such as a history of alcohol or other substance abuse. A healthy lifestyle with plenty of fresh fruit and vegetables, along with moderate exercise can go a long way to help keep dementia symptoms at bay.

Brain Imaging

Brain scans are often used for diagnosing dementia once other simpler tests have ruled out other problems. They are used to check for evidence of other possible problems that could explain a person's symptoms, such as multiple small strokes or a brain tumor. For instance, a "CT" scan can be used to check for signs of stroke or a brain tumor. An "MRI" can provide detailed information about the structure of the brain and if certain portions of the brain are shrinking. Finally, "PET" scans can show patterns of brain metabolism activity and if abnormal amyloid-beta proteins, a classic sign of Alzheimer's disease, have been deposited in the brain.

It is important when you notice signs of dementia or are experiencing memory loss in yourself or a loved one – that a comprehensive workup and consideration of all the possible causes are taken into account. The underlying condition just might be reversible! Each person experiences dementia in a unique way. A skilled physician can correctly put the pieces of the puzzle together to form a clear picture of what is going on physically and mentally. Once the puzzle has been solved, a clear path forward can be mapped.

A typical comprehensive workup to search for reversible as opposed to irreversible causes of dementia might include:

- Formal cognitive testing by a licensed psychologist
- Thyroid status
- Vitamin B1, B6, B12 levels
- Vitamin D
- Folic Acid levels
- ESR
- Quantitative CRP
- Lyme Screen and if positive, Western Blot testing
- RPR (followed by FTA if positive)
- HIV
- Homocysteine level
- Comprehensive Metabolic Profile
- Complete Blood Count
- Erythrocyte (red blood cell) magnesium level
- Stool for ova and parasites (if a history of diarrhea, fever or chills exists)
- MRI and MRA of the brain, to include hippocampal volume measurements

- Assessment for Major Depression (so-called pseudo-dementia of depression)
- Review of current prescription and over-the-counter medications (some cause the symptoms of dementia)
- History of alcohol or other substance abuse
- Neurology evaluation for other conditions (e.g., Parkinson's disease, normal pressure hydrocephalus, tumor, etc.)

If all of these tests/evaluations are negative, measures of amyloid-beta in the brain (for example, an Amyvid PET Scan).

SEVEN

The Road to Diagnosis: One Patient's Story by Bruce Alan Kehr, M.D.

In sickness and in health, each of us manifests unique characteristics. A good doctor is a "medical detective," leaving no stone unturned to get to the bottom of what's wrong, and then how best to treat it. An example of this principle is the story of "Sharon" (not her real name) who came to see me with complaints of memory loss.

Several months ago, Sharon's daughter called my office to see if an appointment with me might be helpful for her mother. Her mother has recently begun having trouble remembering basic things like her granddaughter's name and would park her car in a neighbor's driveway after confusing their house for her own. She wasn't sure if this was just a part of her mother "getting old" or if there might be something medically wrong. I encouraged her to bring her mother into the office for a workup. I assured her there were simple tests that could determine if it might be a more serious problem, and depending on what we uncovered, there would be treatments and steps she and her mother could take to help manage a disease, should one be diagnosed.

The "Work Up"

I met with Sharon and her daughter and took a careful history of her concerns with memory loss, as well as the other worrisome factors her daughter had noticed. I then used a screening test called the MoCA to test Sharon for cognitive impairment, and the results revealed that significant mental impairment was present. I then went through the possible diagnostic tests for dementia (including Alzheimer's Disease), that we could perform to obtain further diagnostic clarity.

I also recommended she get an MRI of her brain to check for any physical problems. Finally, I ordered a number of blood tests to check her nutritional status and overall health. As discussed previously, some nutritional deficiencies and other physical and mental factors can cause signs of dementia and may be reversible.

The Diagnosis

Sharon's blood tests turned out to be normal, and her MRI of the brain did not reveal physical problems like constricted arteries (called ischemic small vessel disease), tumors, normal pressure hydrocephalus, or stroke. Given the results of these tests and the fact that Sharon's memory problems had been worsening rapidly over the past year, and that this rapid progression was not typical of Alzheimer's Disease, I ordered a specialized PET Scan (brain imaging test) that confirmed high levels of a protein called amyloid-beta. These abnormal proteins indicate that Alzheimer's Disease is present, and, sadly, this diagnosis was now confirmed. It is worth mentioning that this type of rapid progression is not typical of Alzheimer's Disease, but is the subject of scientific research. In the context of an unusual presentation of memory loss, a PET scan sensitive to detecting amyloid-beta deposits can be quite valuable. We talked through what the diagnosis meant and devised a plan to help her and her family cope.

Sharon's Treatment Plan

I mapped out a comprehensive three-pronged treatment plan tailored to Sharon's unique needs and circumstances. This included a medical approach called MEND along with prescription medication, supportive care from her daughter, and even technology and resources in the community that are designed to help manage daily life and medical care for those suffering from dementia.

MEND

MEND stands for "metabolic enhancement for neurodegeneration." This means improving cell function and chemical processes in our bodies to prevent cognitive decline. MEND helps to prevent or stem cognitive decline and, in some documented cases, has even shown improvement of cognitive function with patients presenting with symptoms of dementia.

The MEND approach for Sharon included:

- Reducing or eliminating simple carbohydrates (processed sugar)
- Reducing or eliminating gluten and processed food
- Increasing her intake of vegetables, fruits, and fresh fish
- Practicing Yoga

- Increasing sleep time
- Meditating for 20 minutes a day
- Adding Melatonin at bedtime
- Increasing Vitamin D3
- Adding fish oil supplements
- Optimizing oral hygiene with an electric toothbrush

Supportive Care

I worked with Sharon's daughter and Sharon to identify some steps and actions they could take to help support Sharon as she copes with the effects of cognitive decline in daily functioning. As Sharon's Alzheimer's was in an early stage, she could independently carry out daily tasks with minimal assistance. However, checks and balances needed to be put in place.

As Sharon usually woke early in the morning, her daughter committed to a 15 to 20-minute telephone "check-in" each morning, and an extended home visit on Sundays. They would ensure she had bathed and had a plan for meals for the day. They would go over a calendar for any appointments for the day and reinforce them with sticky notes on the refrigerator with times and locations. They also posted important cell phone numbers and emergency numbers to the refrigerator. These numbers were also programmed in Sharon's cell phone. I suggested they start to plan for the future to determine how Sharon would like her affairs handled, and by whom, in the ensuing years, should the decline continue.

Technology and Community

I also encouraged them to reach out on the Internet to trusted sources and organizations that work with dementia patients and their caregivers. A wealth of information can be found on the Alzheimer's Association website at www.alz.org.

I also suggested that they may want to participate in a course or connect with the Insight Memory Care center at www.insightmcc.org, which has a whole host of programming for those with declining memory function and dementia. They focus on both the patient and the caregiver and have activities in which both can participate.

Finally, I also pointed them in the direction of Caring Village. In addition to informative articles and checklists found at www.caringvillage.com/resources, Caring Village's mobile app and dashboard can help caregivers, like Sharon's daughter, coordinate the complicated care of chronic disease management.   Learn   more   at   www.CaringVillage.com/landing.

While Sharon and her daughter may not be able to adhere to this treatment plan 100% of the time, I've found that they manage to follow most of it. Sharon is able to accomplish enough of the MEND plan for it to have a healing and positive effect on her mental functioning. In addition, her daughter is learning as much as possible about the disease, and each is utilizing technology and community resources where helpful. With her treatment plan in place and support from her daughter, Sharon is managing and coping with Alzheimer's in the best possible way for her and her family.

EIGHT

Understanding the Stages of Alzheimer's

Now that we have a better understanding of Alzheimer's and how it fits into the Dementia spectrum let's review the stages of Alzheimer's and how it progresses over time. Alzheimer's disease is divided into three stages: mild (early-stage), moderate (middle-stage), and severe (late-stage). Since Alzheimer's disease affects people in a myriad of different ways, each person will experience symptoms – or progress through Alzheimer's stages- in their own unique way.

Mild (Early Stage)

In the early stages of Alzheimer's, a person may still be able to drive and work. Usually, they can maintain their independence and do not require a caregiver's support. However, friends and family will begin to notice some cognitive problems. These include:

- Problems coming up with the right word or name
- Trouble remembering names when introduced to new people

- Having greater difficulty performing tasks in social or work settings
- Forgetting material that one has just read
- Losing or misplacing important objects
- Increasing trouble with planning or organizing [iv]

Moderate (Middle Stage)

A loved one in the Moderate Stage typically requires supportive care. They have increased trouble with communicating their needs and thoughts, performing daily tasks, and memory problems become even more prominent. These include:

- Forgetting events from the past
- Feeling moody and isolating oneself from friends and family
- Forgetting one's address or phone number
- Confusion about where they are or what they are doing
- Trouble controlling one's bladder and/or bowels
- Becoming confused or agitated in the late afternoon, commonly referred to as "sundowning"
- At-risk to wander and become lost
- Personality changes such as suspiciousness and paranoid delusions
- Compulsive behaviors such as hand-wringing or tissue shredding [v]

Severe (Late Stage)

In the final stage of Alzheimer's, one loses the ability to carry out daily activities independently and suffers from significant cognitive impairments. Those in this stage of the disease require full-time care. This can be the most difficult stage for the caregiver, and active consideration of a full-time nurse or placement in a long-term care facility may be best for everyone.

This stage is also characterized by a loss of physical abilities such as walking, swallowing, and bladder and bowel control. There is an inability to bathe and dress without assistance. Awareness of recent events and one's surroundings will be lost. Even the immune system will become weakened, making them more susceptible to infections such as pneumonia and the flu. It is highly recommended during this stage that the caregiver seeks outside supportive care as the burden will become too great for one to take on alone. Find more information on local senior housing and in-home care services by using Caring Village's free directories.

Tips and Resources for Providing Care along the Way

The following tips and resources can help caregivers manage the care of a loved one diagnosed with Alzheimer's disease.

1. **Communicate:** Ensure you listen closely to your loved one's needs and desires for assistance. It may be hard for them to communicate their feelings, so extra time and care is needed. Remember, "Patience is a virtue."

2. **Beware of Isolation:** Keep your loved one involved in activities that they enjoy and can do easily. Stop over to their house and invite a friend or two if possible. Make dinner or just relax and socialize. Socialization and intellectual stimulation delay disease progression.

3. **Check in for Daily Task Activities:** Call every

morning (if possible) to review the day's planned activities and appointments.

4. **Plan for the Future:** In the early stages, you should discuss how your loved would like their medical and financial affairs handled, and by whom when they are no longer able. Consider downloading Caring Village's FREE Financial, Legal, and Estate Planning Checklist at www.caringvillage.com/checklists/financial-medical-legal-estate/ for more information.

5. **Seek Professional and Community Support:** I have listed some resources below, but you may want to check with a local community center for programs for seniors, ask for suggestions from your primary care doctor or psychiatrist, and search on the Internet for an online support group until you find one that feels like a good fit.

6. **Occupational Therapy**: Occupational Therapists are focused on helping your loved one with their activities of daily living (ADLs).

7. **A Centralized Message Board Calendar** – This area will help your loved one retain orientation information, such as the day of the week, date, month, and year. It also reminds them of the day's events, events from the past few days, and upcoming events. It can include important reminders, such as "take your morning meds at 9 AM," "take a bath", "breakfast is in the pink container in the refrigerator", "walk on treadmill for 30 minutes", and "mail phone bill'" to allow the patient to maintain some semblance of independence and self-worth as a contributor to the family.

8. **Use Smart Phone Technology** – Set helpful reminders with audible and/or vibratory alarms that remind your loved one to eat, take medications, and

keep appointments. These devices can be worn on a strap around the neck to prevent patients from misplacing them.

9. **Consider getting a GPS tracker** – In mid or late stages of Alzheimer's you may want to purchase a GPS tracker to bring you peace of mind knowing where your loved one is at all times.

10. **Daily Exercise:** Regular exercise, like regular social activity, can delay the progression of the disease.

How Caregiving Affects You and Your Family

NINE

The Emotional Impact Caregiving Can Have on a Family

Caregiving can weigh heavily on your emotions, physical well-being, and finances. Unfortunately, the impact does not just rest on your shoulders but impacts the entire family.

"My mom and dad both passed away from Alzheimer's over a year ago. My sister and I, along with supportive husband's and our adult children, cared for them at home. We tried to work in taking care of ourselves as much as we could. Our dad had very combative and angry Alzheimer's and caring for them took a hard toll on us physically, emotionally and mentally. We are still trying to recover."

While every family and situation is different, through our research, we identified three core categories that capture the different emotional challenges a family may experience (source)[11]. Below is a breakdown of each category with actionable suggestions.

3 Ways Caregiving Can Impact the Family

1. Worry, fear, and stress of the disease, ailment, and/or chronic condition of a loved one.

Under certain circumstances, such as cancer or dementia, the unpredictability, misunderstanding, difficult diagnosis, and physical impact on the care recipient can evoke emotions in all family members. These emotions can include fear, sadness, grief, anger, hope, etc. The stress caused by this situation usually bleeds into other areas of one's life, creating secondary stress at work and in family relationships (source)[12]. This kind of stress impacts inter-family relationships causing fights, conflict, and miscommunications. So how can this be avoided?

To create a positive and healthy environment, there are a few proposed methods to inoculate and alleviate the current emotional stress that the family is experiencing including:

- Host a family assessment/meeting on what is needed in order to care for your loved one
- Recognize the hard work of each family members' role
- Openly discuss your emotions without judgment or reaction. Allow people to be heard.
- Use humor in your day-to-day conversations to lighten the load

2. Helping the care recipient deal with the emotional impact of the situation.

Many caregivers feel unprepared because they are thrust unexpectedly into the world and role of caregiving. Learning how to comfort a loved one during a very difficult time and on a subject that is new can be emotionally taxing. Such difficulty can permeate among the family, especially if there is little honesty and infrequent group discussions.

To alleviate this problem, engage your family and learn about your loved one's condition together. Being a cohesive unit, leaning on each, and learning to cope together will make you closer and better able to support each other.

3. Disruptions to family routine, daily living, and dealing with bereavement.

Needing to take time off work, cancel family events, or having to spend a majority of your personal time caring for your loved one can be a disruption to your normal life. That disruption can create a strong sense of resentment directed towards the care recipient, or individual family members depending on their involvement and proximity.

It may sound simple, but to help prevent this from occurring, you need to set a specific schedule for yourself (and family) and follow it. Constantly having day-to-day chaos will have its impact on you, so having a schedule that includes 'me time' will certainly reduce stress.

Many caregivers cope successfully with caregiving and actually experience an improvement in their health/well-being (source)[13]. For many others, however, that is not the case. Being mentally prepared for what may come is necessary. Be open with your family, take action, and engage in a dialogue that includes the three items discussed above.

Want to make it easier to communicate, collaborate, and coordinate your loved one's care? Check out the Caring Village dashboard and mobile app and find out how we're making caregiving easier, safer, and less stressful. Visit Caringvillage.com to learn more!

TEN

Keeping Your Marriage Strong Through Caregiving

"My elderly mother lives with us. For the most part, it is a blessing having her there--but lately, it has become a real stress on our marriage.

For example, my Mom doesn't think I treat my husband as I should. She is used to traditional gender roles and thinks that my husband should have to do nothing beyond work his job and occasionally cut the grass. Our marriage works for us, and we are both happy, but lately, I'm starting to resent him because of her comments."

According to a Caring.com survey, 80% of respondents said caregiving put a strain on their relationship or marriage. The stress of caregiving can quickly become an issue within a marriage because it can affect your daily activities, time, finances, and living space. To keep your marriage strong through the trials and tribulations of caregiving, it's important to understand how caregiving impacts your marriage and what you can do to prevent unnecessary conflict with your spouse.

Caregiving and Marriage

Before we discuss how to prevent conflict within your marriage, you need to understand how caregiving can and does impact your relationships. According to the Mayo Clinic, caregiving can affect your relationship with your spouse by:

- Posing a financial burden
- Cutting into your time together as a couple
- Cutting into the time you have for family matters, such as childcare and housework
- Causing frustration and fatigue
- Causing resentment of the loved one in need or your spouse
- Creating tension or conflict between your spouse and other family members involved in your loved one's care
- Creating more things to disagree about

10 Ways to Keep Your Marriage Strong When Caregiving

Now that you understand how caregiving can impact your marriage, the next step is to take proactive measures to avoid and manage conflict. Below are the top 10 ways to keep your marriage strong, as suggested by numerous experts and articles within the caregiving community:

1. **Acknowledge the issues:** When you start caregiving for an aging parent, recognize the issues

that can come up and discuss strategies on how to manage the upcoming challenges.

2. **Express your concerns:** If your spouse is a caregiver and you are upset, have concerns or other emotions, make sure to schedule time to discuss these issues.

3. **Ask and accept help:** If you are feeling stressed, ask your spouse, family, or friends for help! Here is some additional information on how to get and accept help.

4. **Ask for and grant forgiveness:** We all make mistakes, so don't be afraid to apologize and remember to forgive both yourself and spouse.

5. **Always make time for your relationship:** Put your spouse first. It may be difficult sometimes but always remember to schedule time for just the two of you.

6. **Make decisions together:** If you are making big or small decisions about the care of your aging parent, then do so together. Include your spouse, so they can understand what is happening.

7. **Do activities and events as a family:** If you have to take your aging parent to an appointment, ask your spouse and family to tag along – you can squeeze in more time together this way!

8. **Get outside help as needed:** If the demand is too much for your family, then consider professional care services.

9. **Make communication a priority:** To make this work, you need to have open channels of communication with your spouse. This is the cornerstone of a happy marriage, no matter what.

10. **Be spontaneous and keep the romance alive:** Not everything has to be scheduled. Show your love

with a homemade dinner, a romantic night stroll, or in other personal ways.

Your spouse should always be your number one priority, but life has a way of adding many others to that list. Don't forget to focus on your home life and remember your marriage and family need you too. There will be challenging moments, but being open and honest will go a long way. It will even help to reduce your stress! Act today and discuss these tips with your spouse.

ELEVEN

What is Complicated Grief for a Caregiver?

One of the hardest challenges we will all face is the loss of a loved one. The pain we feel is rooted in the love we had and continue to have based on our memories. Mourning the death of a loved one will affect each of us differently, but it can have a tremendous impact on caregivers. Grief is a natural reaction that our minds and bodies go through. Many people think that grieving ends after the funeral, but grief includes the entire emotional process of coping with a loss, and it can last a long time. A normal amount of grieving gives us the ability to let a loved one go and keep on living in a productive, healthy way. However, caring for someone with dementia, cancer, and other severe chronic conditions can cause what is called complicated grief (CG), which is synonymous with post-traumatic stress disorder.

"Grief is a long journey. It's been 13 months since my father passed and I think finding a new normal has been very hard. Our whole identity was wrapped up in our parent's care. It feels so strange not to think about their care every day."

What is Complicated Grief?

The Mayo Clinic summarizes complicated grief as "painful emotions so long-lasting and severe that you have trouble accepting the loss and resuming your own life." Additional research adds the following characteristics to help you better understand what may initially appear as expected bereavement:

- A powerful sense of confusion
- Immense and unrelenting loneliness
- Sudden and severe panic attacks
- The loss of emotional connection
- Embarrassment or discomfort in expressing grief
- Strong and unshakable sense of destructive guilt
- Hostile behavior that is uncontrollable
- Seeking drugs, alcohol, or other ways to escape reality
- Inability to carry out daily tasks or take on responsibilities
- Suicidal thoughts or feelings of worthlessness

This condition is often mistaken for depression. However, complicated grief is different, as the feelings that those with CG experience don't lessen over time. The death experienced creates a significant divergence of what has occurred from adapting to the new reality.

The Prevalence of Complicated Grief

Complicated grief is a real thing. It is being written about more frequently, and Columbia University even has a program dedicated to studying its impact and ways to cope with it. In one article in Psychology Today, those experiencing CG will "interminably bounce back and forth through the stages of grief without resolution. Research findings show that their brains process grief differently from those who are able to resolve the loss of a loved one. The difference seems to be in the style of yearning their lost loved ones and in hopelessness for the future that prevents them from sufficiently working through the grieving process."

It is expected that 20% of bereaved caregivers will experience severe depression and/or complicated grief as a result of the loss of their loved one. This is a significant percentage of our caregiving population, making this topic all the more important to be open about and raise awareness.

How to Treat Complicated Grief

Knowing about what CG is will help you identify symptoms and take steps to address what is a serious health risk for yourself. If you or a loved one is experiencing this serious condition, you should immediately mobilize your support network by contacting your family and friends. Although it is a struggle, you need to talk about your feelings and acknowledge the new reality of today by remembering your loved one and moving forward with your life.

We will all experience loss and need to prepare ourselves for what may come. Life does go on even in the most difficult of times. You should take this topic seriously and seek professional help and guidance as needed.

How to Prepare to Be a Caregiver

TWELVE

Four Things You Should Consider Before Becoming a Family Caregiver

Family caregivers are the backbone of long-term care for many aging seniors in the United States. While it can save you money compared to other forms of long-term care, the job of caregiver comes a lot of responsibility. When deciding if becoming a caregiver is the best option for you and your loved one consider the following:

- Can you make the time commitment?
- Can you make the financial commitment?
- Can you handle personal care tasks for your loved one?
- Do you have a support system?
- Can You Make the Time Commitment?

Did you know that family caregivers spend an average of up to 24 hours per week on care? If you are working full time, it may require taking time off to fulfill your caregiver responsibilities. Average time spent on caregiving doubles to around 44 hours per week if you are caring for your spouse or partner. Can you take time off of work in order to care for your loved one? 6 in 10 caregivers say they need to make workplace accommodations—cutting hours, taking a leave of absence, receiving a warning about performance or attendance, etc. Also, consider how this time commitment will impact your family.

Can You Make the Financial Commitment?

Depending on the needs of the person you are caring for, caregiving can be expensive. Make sure to take the time to reflect on your own financial situation.

Can You Handle Personal Care Tasks for Your Loved One?

Caring for your loved one can be manageable in the beginning. However, their care needs may increase as time goes on. For example, later stages of Alzheimer's and Parkinson's disease causes individuals to lose more of their independence and ability to take care of themselves. Even if they don't have a chronic condition, as seniors age, they may lose the ability to perform their activities of daily living—routine activities we do every day like bathing, dressing, feeding, grooming, and toileting. 40% of family caregivers find personal care to be the most difficult part of their caregiving responsibilities (source)[1]. Many families opt to hire a professional caregiver if their loved one's care needs exceed what they can handle on their own.

Do You Have a Support System?

"My mother-in-law has dementia, and my father-in-law has something going on as well. Two years ago their doctor said they both need 24/7 care. Both refused to leave their home or to have in-home assistance. Fast forward two years and a lot of arguing....in-home care started and ENDED this week on just the start of the 3rd day. This was with supervision! The adult children were taking shifts and were there at every visit (two 3 hour shifts each day) in an effort to get this new routine working. The siblings can't continue the weekly (more often daily) visits to their parents' house to literally take care of everything that a normal home needs to have done. They have jobs, their own lives, and families. The in-laws won't anyone other than their children to anything. Daily laundry from constant soiled bedding and clothing. Grocery shopping, meds, cleaning, dog care, meals, etc. They can't continue down this road. Something has to give!"

It's important to identify those around you that would be willing to help with Caregiving activities. Which family members and friends would be willing to help?

In addition to family and friends, there may be senior services in your local community, such as transportation and daycare. Respite care is also provided by volunteer organizations such as the Senior Corps and the National Volunteer Caregiving Network. In addition, you can reach out to support staff at the hospital who are in charge of your loved one's case or discharge planning. Families who reach out to these essential support staff can have a guide help them through the difficult journey of caregiving.

Having a support system available to you can help reduce your chances of experiencing caregiver burnout. Think about it: how can you give your loved one the best care possible if you're not at your best?

When to Consider Professional Help

When the going gets tough or when your loved one's care needs exceed what you can handle, you may need to hire a professional. Many families resort to hiring a caregiver from a home care agency—which can cost thousands and thousands of dollars each year. Costs generally range anywhere from $20-24 per hour depending on where your loved one lives.

With eCaregivers, you can work directly with private caregivers to find affordable home care near you. Many of the caregivers on eCaregivers charge rates much lower than an agency—allowing your loved one to receive the most amount of care for less. You can sign up for your free 7-day trial on their website.

Reviewing Your Options

We recommend that you take a look at the current state of your finances and prepare all necessary financial and legal documents for seniors before making a decision. Consider the impact of being a family caregiver will have on work and your social life. See who is in your village for respite care to prevent caregiver burnout. Often, families may choose to care for their loved one until their level of care exceeds what they can handle. What has worked for you? Let us know!

THIRTEEN

How to Find Caregiver Training

Not sure how to do basic hygiene tasks, first aid, or toileting for aging adults? Family caregivers are exposed to new challenges that often result in reactive training (i.e., going to Google when something happens to learn how to deal with it). However, there are many proactive training centers (both online and in-person) that offer a variety of caregiver training courses. If you're in need of caregiver training, take a look at the available resources listed below and find the best option for you.

Family Caregiving Training - Skills You Can Expect to Learn

The following is a list of 19 skills that you could possibly learn about in caregiving training classes:

1. Caregiver job responsibilities
2. Communication skills
3. Personal care and toileting
4. Basic hygiene and basic infection control
5. Emergency procedures

6. Measuring vital signs and documentation
7. Understanding abuse and neglect
8. Stroke care
9. How to assist in Activities of Daily Living (ADLs)
10. Maintaining a clean, safe, and healthy environment
11. Alzheimer's, dementia, and memory care
12. Safety, fall prevention, and first aid
13. Nutrition and meal preparation
14. Exercise and maintaining mobility
15. Infection prevention and control
16. Managing medications and prescriptions
17. Handing difficult behaviors
18. Managing caregiver stress
19. End-of-life care

How to Find Caregiver Training in Your Area

As we said earlier, many of the skills learned are the same required of at-home professional care aids. Below is a list of where you can find training opportunities. If you don't find what you are looking for here, be sure to research directly with your state's Department of Aging. Some additional options include:

Caregiver Training University

The Caregiver Training University site offers training for those wanting to be certified professional caregivers. These skills are applicable to family caregivers, as well. There cost associated with these trainings is roughly $59.

Alzheimer's Association Care Training
At ALZ.org you can find online training options and e-learning workshops that provide training in dementia care. There may be a cost associated with some of the online

courses (around $25-$30). The free e-workshops are available on-demand.

The Institute for Professional Care Education
The Family Learning Center is an online training resource containing over 50 courses created for individuals who are providing care for their loved ones. You can request a free demo to learn more about the online training courses before purchasing them. There is a cost associated with these trainings.

Free Resources Available
In addition to paid trainings, there are free resources available such as:

1. Family Caregiving Alliance: Practical Skills Training for Family Caregivers. This is an overview of the day-to-day, hands-on strategies and skills caregivers need to maintain a frail older or chronically ill individual at home.
2. Health in Aging: Eldercare at Home: Caregiving How-Tos. This site provides guidance and training on common caregiving issues.

Do your research to find out the best option for you. Taking a few minutes to get trained today will help you provide the best care possible.

FOURTEEN

Getting Your CPR and First-Aid Training

"Everyone should know CPR and what to do if someone is choking. It can save lives. That said, using CPR will depend on the situation. If the person whose heart has stopped is very old, CPR can break ribs and puncture the lungs. The bones of people advanced in years (say, 90 and older) can be quite frail. If circulation fails in these people, there needs to be consideration of their final directives. If a living will, or a DNR order are in place, one may opt against doing CPR.

Would I do CPR on a very frail older person who has a living will or DNR order? No. But I would still learn how to do CPR so I might be able to help others."

In any emergency, you will want to be as prepared as possible.

Training in CPR and general first-aid will give you the basic skills you need to know for how to react and read a situation. Find out more about what CPR and first-aid training classes entail and where you can attend these trainings.

What are CPR and First-Aid Trainings?

CPR stands for cardiopulmonary resuscitation (CPR) – a trainable technique that is extremely useful in multiple types of emergencies (heart attacks, near drowning, etc.). You will use CPR when someone's breathing or heartbeat has stopped.

First-aid training may include CPR training, but in general, you will also learn:

* How to assess an emergency
* How to identify what is required for the person in need
* General skills to control bleeding, cuts, and other lifesaving techniques
* How to read signs of a heart attack, stroke, etc.
* And most importantly, when to dial 911

Where Can I Get Trained in CPR and/or First-Aid?

You will want to research organizations in your area that offer in-person or online classes. These trainings may have a fee associated with them, but there are also free options. Below are three prominent organizations that offer training:

* American Heart Association
* The American Red Cross
* National Safety Council

Training for an uncertain future just may help save someone's life. In addition to training, you will also want to have a fully prepped first-aid kit available. Remember, if you are facing an emergency, you should call 911 even if you feel confident in your abilities. The first-responders are medically trained to handle many scenarios.

FIFTEEN

What to Expect as a Caregiver for Someone with Dementia

As we mentioned previously, there are 47.5 million people worldwide currently living with dementia. As the population ages, we will all deal with dementia in some way, as a child of a parent diagnosed, as a friend, loved one, or spouse.

"My grandmother has dementia and constantly asks about her mother, siblings, and husband who have all been deceased for quite some time. At first, we were telling her they had passed away, now we almost try to avoid that subject.

She also lives with her son, but many times thinks he is her husband. Because of this, she gets upset when he is running errands outside the home or visiting friends, because she believes 'her husband' is off somewhere with an imaginary girlfriend."

As a caregiver of someone with dementia, the three main

areas in which to prepare yourself are patience, flexibility, and communication.

Patience

As a caregiver, you can expect that someone with dementia will have problems thinking and remembering what seems like normal tasks or behaviors. This can cause sincere frustration for your aging loved one. This is where patience becomes extremely important. To be patient and help your loved one, use the suggested tips below:

- **Allow for extra time for regular activities:** you need to anticipate that everything will take a little bit longer than usual. Plan your day to include a few extra minutes for each task.
- **Create a routine:** put as much of a routine schedule in place as possible. This will help make the day-to-day less confusing for your loved one.
- **Offer choices and options:** if you are able, provide different options for the day-to-day activities like what to wear, what to eat, or where to go walking. Giving two (maximum three) options will give your loved one some autonomy in decision-making while still helping make things simple.
- **Keep the instructions simple:** give clear, step-by-step instructions when needed. Take your time in order to avoid confusion or frustration.

Flexibility

Dementia is a progressive disease, so you can expect the symptoms and ability to remember or think clearly to decline over time. Be flexible each day, as it may be very different from the day before or the day after. It's important not to become too comfortable. Make sure you keep your eye on your loved one and to put greater supervision in place as the disease progresses. The disease can progress in three stages:

- **Mild Dementia** – some difficulty remembering words, retaining new information, and some behavioral changes.
- **Moderate Dementia** – progressive changes in behavior, cognition, judgment, and general ability to do daily tasks.
- **Severe Dementia** – extensive memory loss, extreme mobility impairment, and other serious needs that require constant care.

You also need to be comfortable asking for help and trying different methods to help care for your loved one.

Clear Communication

Being patient and flexible is critical when communicating with someone affected by dementia. Some tips on how to communicate are:

1. Let the person finish speaking, don't interrupt.
2. Set a positive tone for the conversation and let them communicate at their own pace.
3. Don't criticize or correct.
4. Remain calm and don't let your emotions take control.
5. Be respectful and talk to them as an adult, but be clear and mindful of your pace.

Caring for a loved one with dementia is a challenging job. You need to be aware of how dementia will affect you as the care-giver. Keep in mind how much patience, flexibility, and clear communication will be required daily. Don't forget to give yourself a break and take time for yourself.

SIXTEEN

How Do You Communicate with Someone Who Has Alzheimer's Disease?

Communicating with someone diagnosed with Alzheimer's can be challenging and often create frustration. However, communication is possible if you remain patient, avoid distractions, avoid pointing out mistakes, utilize nonverbal communication, and keep it simple. Read about these tips in more detail below.

5 Tips to Communicate Effectively

Be Patient

When communicating with someone with Alzheimer's, make sure to prepare yourself before entering into a conversation. You need to remain patient and know that it may become challenging. Do not raise your voice, show stress, or demonstrate frustration. Allow your loved one to take their time. Remember to listen and do not interrupt.

Avoid Distractions

Take away the distractions by having the conversation away from competing sights and sounds. You can do this by using a quiet room in the house (like a den or bedroom), so the attention is focused on you and not the TV, the cars driving by, or other background noise. Doing so will at least create a clear pathway for talking.

Avoid Pointing Out Mistakes

You can easily get off-topic or lose someone's attention if you point out a mistake or correct something he or she said. Avoid this mistake and avoid arguing with your loved one.

Utilize Nonverbal Communication

Communication uses both verbal and nonverbal messaging. Try to use visual and nonverbal cues (i.e., hand gestures, facial expressions, etc.) to get your message across.

Keep the Conversation Simple

Depending on where the disease is in its progression, you may need to keep your sentences short and to the point. Eventually, as it progresses, you may need to keep your questions to yes or no answers. In addition, breakdown larger concepts into smaller, easier-to-understand talking points. For example, if you need to discuss a new medication – consider all of the items you need to communicate: the name of the medication, its purpose, why it's happening, when it needs to be taken, how often, etc. Break down each of this and take time messaging it.

There will come a time when the person appears to no longer be able to do "complex tasks" such as brushing their teeth. This difficulty happens because there are many steps to doing this, and the person may not know how to start or forgets some of the steps. Breaking down multi-steps tasks can be helpful. For example, "I am going to help you brush your teeth. Let's take the cap off the toothpaste. Now turn on the cold water. Wet your toothbrush. Put the toothpaste on the brush" , etc. Trying this with tasks a person may see to have forgotten, can help them be more functional for a more extended period of time.

Remember not to take any issues or comments said personally. By being patient and showing respect to your loved one, you can set the tone for the conversation.

How Technology Can Help

SEVENTEEN

The Benefits of Coordinated Calendars for Caregivers

"My sister and I are struggling with juggling the caregiving schedule. We both live an hour away from our mom and are looking for a way to share a calendar and a To-Do List. We just need to be able to look at the caregiver schedule and check in on our To-Do List."

Coordinating schedules among your caregiving team can be a real challenge. Think about how difficult it is to stay on top of your own calendar as a Caregiver with work, family, and other social responsibilities! Find out how the use of a coordinated calendar amongst a group of caregivers can save time and energy, help you avoid mistakes and miscommunications, and ultimately reduce stress for everyone involved.

6 Ways Coordinated Calendars Help Caregivers

Maintaining a coordinated calendar among a group of Caregivers helps you to:

1. Stay organized and informed collectively
2. Ensure responsibilities and appointments are evenly distributed across the team
3. Request help with a given task from within your trusted circle
4. Communicate changes or additions easily and effectively to an entire group
5. Reduce errors and missed appointments
6. Save time and energy

If you implement a coordinated calendar now, you will immediately see relief for all of those involved, including better-coordinated care for your aging loved one. How can you do this? Well, there are several options including, for example:

- A shared Google calendar that everyone can access
- A free online calendar, such as the one offered by Lotsa Helping Hands, that supports the Alzheimer's Association Care Team Calendar
- The Caring Village dashboard and mobile app

Caring Village's easy-to-use dashboard and mobile app include a customizable calendar that will help you coordinate schedules and avoid missed appointments. This feature, in combination with many others, will give you peace of mind knowing that your loved one is being well cared for.

EIGHTEEN

The Top 10 Caregiving Blogs for Caregivers

Being a Caregiver can be tough, and unfortunately, life doesn't slow down to give you time to learn how to care for someone you love. This is why caregiver blogs, which provide resources and information (often from other past or present caregivers and/or industry professionals) can be extremely helpful in navigating your caregiving journey. Below is a list of the top caregiving blogs online including Caring.com, The Caregiver Space, Transition Aging Parents, The Caregiver's Voice, Care-Giving.com, EldercareABC, eCareDiary, Daily Caregiving, Caring for Parents Made Easy, and Caring Village's own resource section.

Caring.com:
https://www.caring.com/blogs
Caring.com is a leading online destination for those seeking information and support as they care for aging parents, spouses, and other loved ones. Their mission is to help the helpers. They equip family caregivers to make better decisions, save time and money and feel less alone — and less stressed — as they face the many challenges of caregiving.

The Caregiver Space:

http://thecaregiverspace.org/

The Caregiver Space provides a safe and open space—at no cost— where visitors can be real about what it's like to care for someone dealing with a serious disability or illness. Use their community forums to ask questions, share experiences, get real answers, or just get things off your chest.

Transition Aging Parents:

http://www.transitionagingparents.com/blog/

Transition Aging Parents is a blog written by Dale Carter, a respected voice for adult children of aging parents. Since facing her own mother's health/life crisis in 2008, Dale has established herself as a voice of reason, as she has traveled around the country from the Midwest to Atlanta, through Florida and New York City. She shares her message of how to approach any change or crisis in your aging parent's life with clarity and confidence. Since immersing herself with authors and experts in the field of gerontology, she has expanded her reach to adult children across this country. She wants to now show you how to guide your aging parent(s) so they can thrive and find joy in every stage of their life.

The Caregiver's Voice:

http://thecaregiversvoice.com/blog/

Founded in 1998 by Brenda Avadian, MA, TheCaregiversVoice.com serves family caregivers and professionals who work with adults with cognitive impairment or dementia caused by Alzheimer's, stroke, related illnesses, or trauma.

CareGiving.com:

http://www.caregiving.com/articles/blogged/

Denise M. Brown launched CareGiving.com in 1996. The site features the blogs of family caregivers, weekly words of comforts, weekly self-care plans, daily chats, a Community Caregiving Journal, free webinars, and daily chats.

EldercareABC:
http://www.eldercareabc.com/
The 'ABC' in EldercareABC stands for 'About Being Connected.' So come in, get connected, and have your say about what information you need. Most importantly discover a group of people that are here to support you and who you can support in your own way.

eCareDiary:
https://www.ecarediary.com/BlogsHome.aspx
eCareDiary is a web community created based on the founders' experiences as caregivers for their parents who were diagnosed with chronic illnesses such as Parkinson's, Type II diabetes, and dementia. Having backgrounds in the healthcare system, they found coordinating long term care to be difficult and frustrating because of the lack of good resources available online. They created eCareDiary.com as a centralized place to help families with care coordination by offering comprehensive online tools, expert content, and resources.

DailyCaring:
http://dailycaring.com
DailyCaring is for the 43.5 million adult family caregivers who care for someone 50+ years of age. They're perfect for family caregivers who use the Internet to find solutions for day-to-day challenges, help with important care decisions, and advice on how to plan for the future. They also cater to help professionals in the aging care industry.

Caregiving for Parents Made Easy:
http://www.caregivingmadeeasy.com/
Caregiving for Parents Made Easy is a site designed to give

you some tips and tricks for navigating the caregiver role. If you're new to caregiving, this site provides places to turn for caregiving resources, as well as general resources for older adults.

Caringvillage.com:
https://www.caringvillage.com/
Caring Village is a caregiving assistance platform that makes caring for an older loved one safer, easier, and less stressful. The Caring Village suite of easy-to-use mobile apps, interactive dashboard, and marketplace allows families to easily communicate, collaborate, and coordinate caregiving activities for their loved ones. With insightful content and preparedness checklists, Caring Village helps provide you with all the information you need to be the best Caregiver you can be.

NINETEEN

The Best Caregiving Podcasts

Are you looking for some quick advice as a family caregiver? Consider listening to a caregiving Podcast. Podcasts have become a great way to listen to the stories of others and learn new things, all at the convenience of the listener. The top caregiving podcasts out there today are Your Caregiving Journey, Dave, the Caregiver's Caregiver, Life is a Sacred Journey, Agewyz, Caregiver SOS, and Caregivers' Circle.

Six Great Caregiving Podcasts

Your Caregiving Journey:

https://www.caregiving.com/listen/

Your Caregiving Journey, with Denise Brown of Caregiving.com, delves into discussions about caregiving situations. Each week, the podcast discusses a topic related to the challenges of caring for a family member or friend. Some recent topics include: policy updates, balancing caregiving and work, and staying positive about money.

Dave, the Caregiver's Caregiver:

http://www.davethecaregiverscaregiver.com/uplifting-interviews/

Dave, The Caregiver's Caregiver, along with his co-host, Adrienne Gruberg, interview different guests each week. Recent topics include incontinence, the right to live or die, and connecting in the land of dementia.

Life is a Sacred Journey:

http://www.blogtalkradio.com/lifeisasacredjourney)

"Life is a Sacred Journey" is designed to share with caregivers and others the many aspects of aging. Micheal Pope, CEO, believes that everyone must contribute if change is to come about. Recent topics include a Caribbean adventure for family caregivers, dismantling ageism, and coping with the daily stress of caregiving.

Agewyz:

http://agewyz.com/podcast-library/

Caregiving guru Jana Panarites engages with unsung heroes — people caring for family members, friends, and relatives amid the demands of their own lives – plus experts in the field of aging and people using film, theater, and other media to creatively address major health issues, foster dialogue, and challenge widespread assumptions about aging. Recent topics include Autism, Alzheimer's, and caring for aging parents.

Caregiver SOS:

http://caregiversos.org/caregiver-sos-podcasts/

Hosted by nationally recognized gerontologist Carol Zernial and veteran broadcaster Ron Aaron, and featuring author/psychiatrist Dr. James Huysman PsyD, LCSW, Caregiver SOS On Air explores issues important to caregivers. Recent topics include: Looking for the right place for your loved ones, are you cut out to be a caregiver, and women wonder.

Caregivers' Circle:

http://webtalkradio.net/internet-talk-radio/caregivers-circle/

Caregivers' circle is a great conversation focusing on the diverse aspects of caregiving. This podcast explores the unique and universal issues that all types of caregivers face, whether the caregivers are adult children looking after their senior relatives, individuals caring for someone with a terminal or chronic illness, seniors caring for adult children with disabilities, or even extended families providing support and care for a family member with a mental health challenge. Recent topics include: Finding life's sweet spots, caregiving guilt, and mental illness.

Happy Healthy Caregiver:

http://happyhealthycaregiver.com/podcast/

This podcast, hosted by Elizabeth Miller, is focused on sharing advice on how to be happy and healthy while caring for others. Her website, HappyHealthyCaregiver.com is a great resource for family caregivers who feel isolated and overwhelmed by all their responsibilities and want help integrating caregiving with their life.

Check out the podcasts listed above and let us know if there are any that we have missed.

TWENTY

The Most Useful Non-Medical Apps for Seniors

Did you know there are more than two million apps available today? These apps provide a variety of services related to health, well-being, entertainment, and much more. We did some research on the most useful apps for seniors and narrowed it down to the top four below. These are non-medical apps available for smartphones and tablets that are consistently ranked in the top three or four of multiple technology review websites. Take a look at each one and share with an aging loved one.

Top 4 Most Useful Non-Medical Apps for Aging Adults

Check out the apps listed below and see if any are the right fit for you.

Magnifying Glass with Flashlight
https://itunes.apple.com/us/app/magnifying-glass-flashlight/id908717824?mt=8
The Magnifying Glass and Flashlight with flashlight (LED Torch Light) can handle all your fine print reading needs. Simply turn on the magnifier and watch as it autofocuses the

text while providing you the ability to zoom in/out further. Finally, you'll see everything big and clear.

Red Panic Button

https://play.google.com/store/apps/details?id=uk. ucsoftware.panicbuttonpro&hl=en

Red Panic Button is designed to improve the lives of all citizens by offering them a higher degree of security in our society. As a mobile device, the application offers users safety guidance in unknown environments (using a GPS option) and helps people feel confident and safe when moving or working. You just have to set a panic number or mail address, and the phone will send a message containing your location, determined using the fine GPS-based or coarse GSM-based coordinates.

Audible

https://www.audible.com

Audible allows you to listen to your books wherever you are with their free app—at home, in the car, at the gym. Even if you switch devices, you'll never lose your place. Home to a library of over 180,000 audiobooks, podcasts, and Audible cChannels, with complete customization of your listening experience. Instantly begin your 30-day free trial today and stream your first audiobook free!

Shopwell

http://www.shopwell.com/mobileapp

Shopwell tells you what's in the food you're buying at the grocery store and offers suggestions for new foods to try that fit with your lifestyle. Simply scan any item in the grocery store, and the app will give you all of the information about that product. Create a profile with your food interests, and Shopwell will suggest similar products that best match your interests right in the store you're standing in.

How to Formulate Your Caregiving Plan

TWENTY-ONE

How to Formulate Your Caregiving Plan

No matter where you are in your journey as a caregiver, something all family caregivers need to establish is a caregiving plan of action. Get started today on creating your own caregiving plan with these six steps.

How to Create Your Caregiving Plan in Six Steps

Step 1: Prepare Yourself and Your Family

There are important things to consider when you start caring for an aging loved one or someone in need of assistance, such as:

- Can you manage the time commitment necessary? (Be honest with your answer.)
- Can you manage the financial commitment using your own finances?
- Can you handle the personal care tasks for your aging loved one or do you need/want professional help?
- Do you have a support system – i.e., a network of

others that can help you, such as family members, friends, neighbors, professionals?

Step 2: Evaluate Your Aging Loved One's Needs
You should understand exactly what your loved one will need as you begin to care for them. To do that, these questions will help organize your thoughts:

- What care is needed? What will your role be in providing care? Will you provide the care or do you need to organize professional in-home care?
- When and how long will the care be needed – daily, weekly, or 24-hour care? Is this a short-term or long-term care situation?
- Do you have the training needed to support your aging loved one?

Step 3: Open Up Communication with All Stakeholders

Open and honest communication will be extremely valuable for you, your family, and your aging loved one. Difficult topics to communicate about may include: decisions about finances, the need for others to help with caregiving, changes in health and wellness, decreased mobility, transitions of care, and more. The first place to start is to discuss the future of care with your aging loved one. Next, you need to have an open dialogue with all of your family members and those within your support network to establish the next steps and put them into action.

Step 4: Form Your Caregiving Team

Putting together your care team will not be done overnight. You will need to take practical and thoughtful steps towards assembling and coordinating a team that is focused on one mission: to provide the best care possible for your loved one. Not sure how to assemble your team or who to include? Be sure to read the next section of this book and check out Caring Village's easy-to-use mobile app and dashboard.

Step 5: Establish Your Plan

With your support network established, and a deep understanding of your aging loved one's needs – you can begin working on your Caregiving plan. To help get you started, review our Caregiving 101 Checklist in the Resources section of this book.

Step 6: Implement Your Plan

Once you've worked your way through the checklist and laid out your plan, get to work on it right away. Have regular check-ins with your loved one and your caregiving team. Don't be afraid to adjust your plan based on new information and day-to-day changes.

The six steps listed above are a great starting point. As you embark on your caregiving journey, please revisit CaringVillage.com for helpful articles, checklists, and other frequently updated resources. Send us your questions and comments, and remember you are not on this journey alone!

TWENTY-TWO

How to Communicate with an Aging Loved One About Their Care

"My grandfather has middle stage Vascular Dementia due to a stroke, and I'm wondering how best to communicate with him. I don't want to confuse him by using complicated language, but I also don't want to talk down to him. He was very intelligent, and he can still tell when someone is talking down to him."

Is your aging loved one at the point where they need additional care? If you are (or will be) their primary caregiver, you need to know how to effectively communicate with them about certain difficult subjects about the future.

One of these subjects is how they would like to be cared for as they age. For the caregiver, this can sometimes be a frustrating and painful conversation to have, especially if your loved one is resistant or unwilling to accept or face reality. Below are some best practices to help you get through these important discussions with your loved one.

How to Connect, Listen, and Communicate with a Loved One About Their Care

Keep the following in mind when communicating with a loved one about their care:

1. **Know why you are having the conversation in the first place.** Before getting started, determine why you are meeting and what you are going to discuss. Is this what you want or what they need? These simple questions can often create conflict if not immediately addressed.

2. **Be a good listener and remember that this is a difficult subject.** This is the time when you need to be quiet and listen to find out what matters to your loved one. By listening, you are letting your loved one know that you care about their feelings and taking the opportunity to learn more.

3. **Engage using both emotion and logic.** This is an emotional and difficult topic. Your loved one may be scared, angry, confused, or in denial, preventing them from accepting the truth. Before starting the conversation, ask yourself, "How would I advise my friend in this same situation?" This is a helpful technique to put you in the right frame of mind. Find the right emotional connection when talking with your loved one. If they are scared, start by telling them you love them and describe clearly what is needed for their health.

4. **Be ready for anything.** The conversation may get off course for any number of reasons so be prepared for that. Use your best judgment while you're in the

situation and if things get too emotional, consider pausing and trying again another day.

5. **Have patience and perseverance.** Having a conversation and making decisions about how one wants to be taken care of as they age can be physically and emotionally taxing, so be patient and take your time. This one discussion will likely evolve into multiple discussions until a decision is reached.

Best Practices for Communicating with an Aging Parent

Consider the following when initiating a difficult conversation with your aging parent:

- Write down your objective and stick to it. This will keep you on track in the event the conversation changes if/when the subject becomes emotional.
- Understand your communication style so that you are able to manage your emotions and clearly articulate what you mean.
- Understand your aging parent's communication style (i.e., how do they receive information), so you are prepared and can keep the conversation focused.
- Consider the type of information being shared both from you and from your parent. Your parent may have great ideas or serious concerns and it is important to listen.
- Choose the best environment/location to hold the conversation, so you both feel comfortable and are not interrupted.
- Remember personal style (such as the use of body language, tone of voice, choice of words, speaking) because this can often cause conflict or misunderstanding.
- Keep in mind your pace and word choice. This will

ensure that the message is clear, articulate and on target.

Remember that you are not the first and, unfortunately, will not be the last person to have this type of conversation. Use the suggested tips above to ensure that you're fully prepared and communicate effectively.

TWENTY-THREE

How to Create Your Caregiving Team

Henry Ford said it best: "Coming together is a beginning, keeping together is progress, and working together is success." The value of a team and the success of a team starts at its formation. As a caregiver, you need to know how to create a cohesive and collaborative team of caregivers, supporters, and medical experts.

Creating Your Caregiving Team

To create your caregiving team:

Start with an initial assessment of the situation: Begin by evaluating the who, what, when, where, and why.

- *Who:* Who is the care recipient? Is it a family member, friend, etc.?
- *What:* What help do you need? What are you able to do yourself? What are your strengths? What are your weaknesses?
- *When:* When do you need additional help? How long will you need this help?

- *Where:* Does your loved one live at your house? Does the team need to travel to help? What can the team do remotely?
- *Why:* What is your vision for the team? How would you like others to help you?

Determine the needs of the care recipient: Next, you will need to explain the needs of the care recipient. What support does your loved one need? Will they need medication management? Transportation? Do they require additional help for limited mobility? Do they have any chronic conditions such as Alzheimer's? Do they require professional or medical help?

Identify potential team members: Determine and list out who you think will need to be (or should be) on your caregiving team. This can include:

- Family members (siblings, cousins, spouse)
- Friends
- Neighbors
- Medical support
- Professional caregivers

Create clear role delineation: Defining who does what can be difficult. If you have assessed the situation and determined the needs of your loved one, you can then identify and clearly articulate the roles needed on the team. You may even want to enlist their help in defining the roles in more detail. This will help your family, friends, neighbors, etc., to understand your needs and expectations.

Develop a communication strategy: You can start by having an initial meeting with all those involved to discuss who will do what and then outline the next steps. You should hold regular check-ins with everyone.

Putting together your team (or village) will not be done overnight. You will need to take practical and thoughtful steps towards assembling and coordinating a team all focused on one mission: to provide care for your loved one. One convenient and practical way of implementing and coordinating with your team is with the Caring Village app. This "caregiver planner" app can be used as the command center for all of your caregiving needs and activities. Learn more about it at www.CaringVillage.com.

TWENTY-FOUR

How to Find Caregiver Resources in Your Area

Caregiving is a tough job. As a Caregiver, you're tasked with an entirely different set of responsibilities, sometimes overnight, in addition to your regular daily life. It's stressful, overwhelming, and can become very difficult to manage at times. How do you make it all work? Who can you turn to for assistance?

If you are a Caregiver, you should know that there are several federal, state, and local departments dedicated to providing caregivers with the resources they need. We've provided an overview of some of these organizations below.

National Association of Area Agencies on Aging

The National Association of Area Agencies (N4A) is a conglomeration of the Area Agencies on Aging (AAAs). AAAs were formally established in the 1973 Older Americans Act (OAA) as the "on-the-ground" organizations charged with helping vulnerable older adults live with independence and dignity in their homes and communities. To locate local area resources, you can use the N4A's searchable database powered by Eldercare.gov. To do this, follow the steps below:

- Visit www.n4a.org
- Enter your city/state or zip code
- Click search

The result of this search will provide a list of available resources in your community with contact information, links to dedicated websites, as well as a brief description. You can locate an Area Agency on Aging (AAA) by using the Administration for Community Living's database powered by the U.S. Department of Health and Human Services. To use ACL, follow the steps below:

- Visit www.aoa.gov/AoA_programs/OAA/ How_To_Find/Agencies/find_agencies.aspx
- Select your state from the drop-down menu
- Choose your county

This search will provide you with a link to the website, as well as contact information for the state aging care office (if applicable), as well as the Area Agency on Aging.

Aging and Disability Resource Center

The Aging and Disability Resource Center (ADRC) provides a single, coordinated system of information and access for individuals seeking long-term services and support. It is an initiative of the Department of Health and Human Services. To use this resource, follow the steps below:

- Visit http://www.adrc-tae.acl.gov/tiki-index.php? page=ADRCLocator
- Click on your state, then select your county

- Once the new window opens, review the available resources

Family Caregiver Alliance's Online Caregiver Support Group

The Caregiver Online Group is an online network and safe space for families and other caregivers of adults with chronic debilitating health conditions to discuss the stresses, challenges, and rewards of providing care for a loved one. To use the online support group, follow the steps below:

- Visit http://lists.caregiver.org/mailman/listinfo/ caregiver-online_lists.caregiver.org
- Subscribe online with your name and email address
- Enter the online community to find support from others and find more personalized resources

First and foremost, remember that you are not alone; there are tons of resources out there if you know where to look. Before you start your research, identify what questions you need answered, what types of resources you need, and who will be the recipient of these resources, you or your loved one. Once you have answered these questions, begin your search and contact the appropriate office(s) for help.

TWENTY-FIVE

What is a Geriatric Social Worker?

If you are looking for someone to help be an advocate for your aging loved one, then you may want to find a geriatric social worker. Geriatric social workers make up about 5% of the nation's 600,000+ social workers. These hard-working individuals can help older adults overcome many challenges and can connect them with vital resources and services. Not sure if you need a social worker or where to start? We've outlined some helpful information about the many services available from geriatric social workers.

What Is Geriatric Social Work?

The field of social work utilizes social theories to understand human problems, to help improve people's lives, and to improve society as a whole. Many who work in this field specialize in particular areas, such as helping children, assisting those with life-threatening problems, or aiding people in overcoming addictions. Geriatric social workers help those above the age of 65 adjust to and cope with problems they may experience. These social workers focus on the unique needs that older adults may experience.

How Can a Geriatric Social Worker Help?

Geriatric social workers are trained to assist the elderly as they deal with a wide assortment of problems, like mental disorders, social problems, financial issues, emotional problems, and health care needs. Geriatric social workers typically perform the following job functions:

- Assessing the needs, strengths, weaknesses, situations, and support systems of elderly clients and patients, in an effort to develop short-term and long-term goals and treatment plans
- Developing treatment plans that are designed to improve the mental health and well-being of elderly clients and patients
- Helping clients and patients adjust to life changes (i.e., illnesses, divorces, debt, death, and/or unemployment)
- Researching and referring elderly clients and patients to resources (i.e., government housing, medical services, Meals-on-Wheels, transportation, and food stamps)
- Helping elderly clients and patients sign up for government assistance (i.e., Medicare)
- Tracking the progress of elderly clients and patients
- Acting as a liaison and advocate for elderly clients and patients
- Arranging social activities and gatherings for elderly clients and patients

There are many places to find professional social workers who provide individual psychotherapy and other forms of mental health assistance, including group therapy and support groups. To find your social worker visit the National Association of Social Workers and search in your area.

TWENTY-SIX

When Should My Parents Move in With Me?

"My mother recently moved in with me. I no longer have my home and am miserable but would never tell her so. I adore her. I'm 48 with a boyfriend and a dog and live alone and LOVE IT that way. I feel like she has other options other than just me, but I do love her deeply, and I don't know what to do."

As the baby-boomer generation reaches retirement and gets older, you may find yourself at a place where you're considering whether or not the time is right for your parent(s) to move in with you. This presents other questions such as: Is my house ready? Is my family ready? Am I ready? And most importantly: Are my parents ready?

According to estimates from the National Alliance for Caregiving, during the past year, 65.7 million Americans (or 29% of the adult U.S. adult population involving 31% of all U.S.

households) served as family caregivers for an ill or disabled relative. The decision to have a parent or parents move in is important and should be made early to help mitigate any unpredictable health or physical changes. The main resources you need to consider are:

- Time
- Finances
- Space
- Relationships

Time

It is essential to begin the conversation early with your parents. Although it's not always an easy conversation to have, it's important to create an action plan that is agreed upon by your parents beforehand. In general, caregiving results in major changes in a family and physical, emotional, social, and financial issues often arise. Creating a harmonious dialogue between you and your parent(s) early keeps the lines of communication open and set a clear understanding of expectations. This will also allow you to prepare for the type of care your parent(s) will need no matter the situation.

Finances

Proper planning will allow you to make spending and budget adjustments within your household. Parents that require care may see cost savings if they move in with their children, depending on the situation. According to a new study conducted by Caring.com, nearly half of family caregivers spend more than $5,000 a year on expenses associated with providing care. Of those spending more than $5,000, 16% are seeing costs of as much as $9,999 while 11% are spending as high as $19,999 and 5% are absorbing out of pocket expenses of as much as $49,999.

In addition, "People in their 50s and 60s are spending a significant part of their money caring for aging parents," says Caring.com Chief Executive Andy Cohen. "People do a good job of saving for their kid's college and their own retirement, but they don't know this is coming."

Coordinate this change with your family and determine who will manage your parent(s) finances, what will happen to their estate, and learn how to manage their property and the new costs you can anticipate. Consult with a financial advisor early and begin saving for these future changes.

Space

Start by asking yourself: is my home designed for this change? Remember, what is normal for you may become extremely challenging for your parent(s). Navigating stairs, bathtubs, handrails, the width of doorways and hallways for wheelchairs become important things to take into consideration. Proper planning of your parent(s) needs will identify and determine what types of assistance they will need, as well as aid you both in time and finances.

Renovation costs can be burdensome so plan ahead since even installing an electric stairlift for moving from floor to floor usually runs about $5,000 to $10,000, depending on the manufacturer. Also, consider any pieces of property that may accompany your parent(s) with this change and how to accommodate them.

Relationships

Are you ready and prepared for this change? It is critical to consider the emotional and psychological energy an aging or infirm parent may require. Consider yourself, your parents, and your children in this decision and involve them from the beginning.

If you decide to suggest this change, be especially mindful of your parents, involve your entire family, and encourage everyone to ask questions throughout the process. If you and your parent(s) decide to move forward with this change, you should first identify any needs they may have, consolidate financial and legal documents, keep track of any immediate or potential health needs, and finally complete the initial assessment checklist to create your action plan.

TWENTY-SEVEN

When is It Time to Hire a Professional Caregiver?

"My mom is 72 now, and we (me and my wife) were taking care of her for the past eight years. Recently my wife had surgery, and I felt uneasy about managing both my mom and my wife's case. I searched for some caregiver services and found an excellent one. Initially, I was not sure if I made the right decision or not, but their service was awesome, and my mom is really feeling comfortable with her caretaker. We are continuing to use their service even after my wife's recovery."

Are you providing care for a loved one in need of assistance? If so, are you trying to find additional help and not sure what that would look like or where to start? Additional help can be found in hiring a professional caregiver. Below are some suggested questions to ask yourself to help evaluate if you need to hire a professional caregiver. These questions will help you conduct your own evaluation of the situation and make the best decision possible.

How to Evaluate When You Need to Hire a Professional Caregiver

To help you best determine if you need to hire a professional caregiver, answer the questions below, starting with 'Does your loved one':

- Want to live at home?
- Require daily medical treatment or attention beyond your expertise?
- Have mobility issues requiring 24/7 support?
- Have a chronic condition impacting his/her memory and general ability to manage day-to-day activities?
- Cause you significant stress and anxiety, ultimately impacting your health?
- Require you to take a significant amount of time off from work?

If you answered "Yes" to one or more of these six questions, then you may want to consider hiring additional help. Hiring a professional caregiver can help not only with providing care for your loved one but can also benefit you by reducing stress and enabling you to remain focused on other priorities in your life such as work and family. The type of support a caregiver can provide at home includes:

- Medication management
- Bathing and general daily support
- Cooking/cleaning
- And much more

Additional Considerations When Hiring a Caregiver

The decision to hire a caregiver can be considered from two different viewpoints: the family caregiver's perspective and the care recipient's perspective. As the family caregiver, the need for hiring a professional caregiver may be obvious since you experience the most significant burden. However, your aging loved one (the care recipient) may not think hiring help is necessary since they are used to you always being there.

If you do decide to hire a caregiver, remember that you are not surrendering nor are you being selfish. In fact, the decision should be in the best interest of your loved one with the goal of providing the best quality care for them. Many people have hired home caregivers based on different needs – from help with the activities of daily living to companionship. So, evaluate your situation, discuss your recommendation with your family and loved one, and make the best choice that helps everyone.

TWENTY-EIGHT

Residential Care Options for Aging Adults

Choosing to move out of your home can be a hard decision. For aging adults, moving into a residential care facility (i.e., nursing home) can be even more challenging. We all want to give our loved ones the option of living at home, but there may come a point where more care is necessary. That's when you may decide to encourage your loved one to move to a residential care facility. Keep in mind that these housing options will differ based on the following:

- if they are required to be licensed or not
- the overall cost
- the population they serve
- other potential factors

The most common types of residential care you can explore in your community are Assisted Living, Care Homes, Independent Living Communities, Nursing Homes, Memory Care, Continuing Care Retirement Communities, and Hospice.

Assisted Living

"I've noticed my dad, who lives alone since my mom died last year, is much more wobbly than he used to be. He is aware of it and really tries to be careful. My mother-in-law, who also lived alone for a year after her husband died, kept tripping on her clunky shoes and falling. She'd trip and fall, and if she didn't break anything (like she eventually did to her hip) but she wouldn't remember falling because of the dementia. Instead, she might complain that her head hurt. So I'd start looking at her through her hair, and sure enough, there would be dried blood where she had banged her head on something and forgotten. She's in assisted living now, and I feel like it's so much safer."

An assisted living facility (or home) can offer a wide range of 24/7 support. The staff at these facilities assume responsibility for your aging loved one's safety and well-being. Some of the common services provided include laundry, housing, transportation, meals, recreational activities, assistance with activities of daily living (ADLs), and even some nursing care. The size of the facility will vary based on location but often have at least ten residents. These types of residences are licensed by the state and in some cases, offer subsidies for low-income seniors.

Care Homes

Similar to Assisted Living Facilities are Care homes, which are also known as board and care homes or residential care homes. While residents at care homes receive assistance with

ADL's, they do not receive skilled nursing or medical care. Typically, this option is good for those aging adults who prefer a more intimate setting, as Care homes tend to be private and much smaller that Assisted Living facilities.

Independent Living Communities

Independent living communities are apartments (or condos) that are age-restricted. This means that the minimum age for a resident is 55 years or older. These communities are exclusive for older adults and typically offer a friendly, social environment, including recreational activities and other general services. The residents usually are in overall good health, so the staff is not providing any additional care or supervision. These are often associated with Continuing Care Retirement Communities (CCRC), which are very similar in purpose and function.

Nursing Homes

In nursing homes, older adults are given round-the-clock care by licensed, skilled nursing staff to fulfill their basic care needs. They provide some medical care but do not provide as much high-level medical care as hospitals. Under medical supervision, nurses carry out non-surgical treatments of chronic diseases. In addition, there are trained speech, occupational, and physical therapists, who support the residents in a variety of ways.

Memory Care

Memory care residential facilities are designed to support older adults with Alzheimer's, Dementia, and other forms of memory issues. You may also hear them referred to as special care units. These units provide 24-hour supervised care (often within an assisted living home). These can be extremely helpful to you and your loved one because they provide a personalized plan to address common emotional, physical, and intellectual concerns associated with memory disorders.

Continuing Care Retirement Communities

While most retirement communities only offer independent or assisted living, CCRC's provide residents with a continuum of care. They include independent living, assisted living, and memory care facilities.

Hospice

Hospice residential care options provide care for those with a terminal illness who need trained, skilled staff to care for them. Those who need hospice care will receive 24-hour nursing care and support from staff specifically trained in hospice care.

As you can see, there are many residential care options available. This means your aging loved one can get the specific care they need. The help and support is out there – so use this as a starting point. Go out and see these facilities for yourself to make a better judgment on what works best for you and your loved one.

Also, if you've done your research and you're still not sure, consider enlisting the help of a Geriatric Care Manager. They are professionals who perform an assessment of a person's mental, physical, environmental, and financial conditions to create a care plan to assist in arranging housing, medical, social, and other services.

How to Care for Yourself While Providing Care

TWENTY-NINE

How to Identify, Prevent, and Reduce Caregiver Stress

"Since June, I have become the full-time caregiver to my mother. She has been in a wheelchair for several years, but until last winter she was able to transfer herself to her chair or bed. Now she can't stand or walk, and we have to use a lift to move her. She also has a tracheotomy but uses a speaking valve to talk. Plus she is on a ventilator at night. All during the summer, my teenage daughter and I took care of her, and now my daughter helps when she can, but she is busy with school too. We have moved into my mother's house, leaving my house and husband to "fend for himself." I have been accused of yelling at my mother when I try to get her to complete therapy or try to get her to follow doctors orders or anything else my mother doesn't want to hear. I feel lost and like I'm losing my mind half the time."

Caring for a family member or a loved one can be both extremely rewarding and emotionally taxing. You need to know the signs of caregiver fatigue and how to proactively prevent stress and potential emotional harm. In order to prevent caregiver stress (the emotional and physical strain of caregiving), you need to know the signs and take measurable steps to prevent it from impacting your health and well-being.

What Are the Signs of Caregiver Stress?

Generally, the signs of caregiver stress (or fatigue) include the following:

- Uncontrollable frustration or anger
- Loneliness
- Physical and/or emotional exhaustion

Any and all of the feelings above can dramatically affect your health and cause unhealthy changes in your diet, mood, stress level, and ability to sleep. If you are a caregiver experiencing any of these symptoms, it is critical that you seek medical care and take time for yourself immediately.

5 Ways to Reduce Caregiver Stress

You can reduce or prevent stress by taking the appropriate time to learn about your parent or loved one's needs before becoming the caregiver. This can include:

1. Researching the illness
2. Understanding the financial aspect of the situation
3. Talking with others
4. Being OK to say 'no'
5. Making time for your own needs

In addition to the list above, creating a routine is essential. With a routine, you will easily notice any sudden changes in your behavior or stress level (caused by a deviation from your routine). Also, don't be afraid to ask for help when you need it. Not asking for help when you need assistance will increase your stress level.

Caregiver stress or fatigue is real and can affect you at any point. It can impact men and women differently, so be proactive and monitor your stress level. About 75% of caregivers who report feeling very strained emotionally, physically, or financially are women. Research shows that people who take an active, problem-solving approach to caregiving issues are more likely to feel less stressed. Follow the tips above and be proactive about your stress. Taking the time to take care of yourself mentally and emotionally will help you to be the best caregiver you can be.

THIRTY

How to Stay Positive as a Caregiver

"My 85-year-old father and his little untrained dog moved into my house in April after my mom passed in January. I have two kids, a husband, work from home, but travel for work often. For the most part, the arrangements have worked for him, but I am having a hard time dealing. I have a really good attitude, but sometimes the situation really gets to me. I need to make sure that I am doing him service and me too."

Do you live your day with a positive outlook? Do you do everything you can to keep your spirits up? Well if you do then we have good news for you – you may live a longer, healthier life as a result. Several recent studies have consistently found that being positive is good for your health. This becomes even more important for those dealing with difficult life challenges, in particular being a family caregiver.

While it may be challenging at times, here are six tips to help you stay positive when you are caring for a loved one.

6 Ways to Remain Positive as a Caregiver

1. **Keep a gratitude journal** – Life is busy, and we can easily forget about all of the good things in our lives, in favor of focusing on the bad. The best way to remind ourselves of the positives in each day is through a gratitude journal. How it works is you write down five things you are grateful for each day. It can be as small as someone holding the door open for you to something bigger, like being thankful for your family and friends. This will capture your daily positives for you to reflect on when needed.

2. **Act happy to feel happy** – Have you ever heard the expression "fake it till you make it"? When you are stressed or having a hard time, put a smile on your face. Smiling, even when you don't feel like it, is scientifically proven to help improve your mood. Take it even further by using positive words to describe your day, week, and when talking about your life in general. If you say, act, and tell yourself happy thoughts, you can start to reframe your outlook on life.

3. **Surround yourself with good people** – Who we spend time with will influence how we feel. Spend time with those people that are positive and supportive. Surround yourself with those loved ones who make you feel good and don't deplete you of energy.

4. **Focus and find energy in your possibilities** – Think about your future opportunities and possibilities. This is very important to prevent you

from getting lost in the daily grind, or focusing on the past. Write down your goals and revisit them often. Keep your focus on the future.

5. **Let your body lead the way** – Your body knows when to take a break. We can all muster up enough energy to get us through a long day, but you need to listen to your body and know when to stop. Rest will give you the energy you need to keep up the positive attitude.

6. **Do something kind** – We often will feel better when we do something good for someone else. So try it out! There are plenty of ways to do something kind: lend a helping hand to someone in need, make a donation, volunteer, spend time with a loved one, and much more. This will help someone else and help you at the same time.

The steps above are some of the many ways to remain positive as a caregiver. We hope you try out at least one of the suggestions above to help you live a more positive life.

THIRTY-ONE

How to Accept Help as a Caregiver

Are you a Caregiver? Have you ever been offered help, really needed it, but instead of accepting it said, "No thanks, I can do it myself?" There are many reasons why accepting help is difficult for some. However, accepting help is one way to prevent caregiver stress. Train yourself to say "Yes" to someone offering assistance by reminding yourself that others can help you and, in many cases, you can actually accomplish more by delegating to others. Remember, you are not a burden if you accept help from others, and it's very important that you take care of yourself and not try to accomplish everything on your own.

Why Caregivers Should Accept Help

Your instinct when being offered help may be to say no. This is not uncommon for reasons such as: wanting to protect your loved one, feeling competitive, concern for your own privacy (or the privacy of your loved one), and a feeling of guilt. To move you from 'no' to 'yes,' keep in mind the following:

- **You are not a burden** - If someone is genuinely offering to help you and/or your loved one, it is okay to accept it. The offer may be specific (i.e., to cook dinner or pick up groceries) or vague enough to allow you to identify what you need assistance with. If the offer is on the table, then you should accept it and just simply say "Yes, thank you." In fact, if you turn down the offer to help, you may be insulting the person offering. Your acceptance may even help that other person feel better because they are providing help to you and the person you are caring for.
- **It's important to take care of yourself** - As a caregiver, it's extremely important to monitor your stress level and to be mindful of your own health and well-being. Accepting help may give you the time you need to focus on your own needs, just as you need to focus on the needs of your loved one. Getting help is not a weakness but an acknowledgment that we can all do more as a coordinated team.
- **You can let go, and still maintain control** - Having someone else's help is not an admission of weakness or a loosening of your control. In fact, having a helpful pair of hands can give you some time to refocus, recharge, and re-evaluate the situation. Your acceptance of help is a recognition of your own capabilities and needs in a positive way. You are still in control when you delegate work.

It may be a challenge for you, but the next time someone offers help, say 'yes'! Take them up on the offer and you may just be surprised at the relief you feel. In the end, the benefit of accepting help is improving your well-being, as well as that of your loved one.

THIRTY-TWO

Caregiving Resources: Daughters in the Workplace

Women make up two-thirds of all family caregivers. A recent survey found that 50% of those female caregivers feel they need to choose between caregiving, working, and parenting. This challenge is felt throughout the caregiving community. According to the Family Caregiver Alliance, the average caregiver is a 49-year-old married, employed woman, caring for her 60-year-old mother who does not live with her. A new program, Daughters in the Workplace, was recently implemented to help start the conversation about how working family caregivers can be better supported in the workplace.

What is Daughters in the Workplace?

Daughter's in the Workplace is a new public education program created by the Home Instead Senior Care company. Daughters in the Workplace offers free resources to family caregivers that are intended to empower the caregiver with strategies. These resources also provide important information to aid her in discussing her needs with her employer, as well as identify caregiving support in the area. Additionally, this program will provide employers with helpful information on what their employee may need or be going through.

How to Access Daughters in the Workplace

To access the many tools available, visit www.caregiverstress.com/stress-management/daughters-in-the-workplace/.   On the website, you can scroll through the many articles and videos available. Topics include:

- When Work Works for You: Identifying What Support You Need as a Working Family Caregiver
- 10 Ways Family Caregivers Can Feel Empowered at Work
- Conversation Starters: How to Talk to Your Employer About Your Caregiver Support Needs

In addition, there is a short quiz to help you answer, "Can you take time off work to care for Mom?" The questions are meant to help you better understand the Family Medical Leave Act (FMLA) which we discussed in some detail in the previous section of this book.

Overall, if you provide care for an aging parent and find it difficult to balance it all, the Daughter's in the Workplace free service may be a helpful resource. Check it out and see for yourself.

THIRTY-THREE

What is Respite Care?

Caregiving is tough and requires a significant amount of time and energy. However, even as a family caregiver, it's important to take breaks – or in other words, "respite." Respite Care can help family caregivers by relieving them of their duties temporarily while ensuring their loved one is receiving safe and professional care. During this time, you can take some 'me' time. Find out more about what Respite Care is, the types of Respite care available, and why you should use it.

Types of Respite Care

Respite care can be found in several different places, including:

Family and Friends: Don't be bashful about asking for help. You can reach out to your immediate family, family friends, and also neighbors, local faith groups, and others within your inner circle. Be sure to plan in advance and provide helpful notes for any friends or family members that will be stepping in for a few hours or days.

Professional At-Home Services: Hiring professional

caregivers can provide relief as well. There are different kinds of in-home care available including: professional skilled nurses, personal caregivers, home companions, and home-makers. Research each of these to find what is right for you. Other unpaid caregivers can also provide in-home services. These individuals will often be trained as a part of a local organization that provides this type of service. For more information about professional home services, check out these resources:

- CareLinx - https://www.carelinx.com/
- Caring.com - https://www.caring.com/local/in-home-care
- Home Team - https://www.hometeamcare.com/
- Honor - https://www.joinhonor.com/

Veteran Respite Care: Respite care for veterans is available through the Geriatrics and Extended care program through the Veterans Administration. You can find more information on this program by clicking here. For those eligible, this service will pay for a person to come to a veteran's home or for a veteran to attend a program to give their caregiver a break.

Community Organizations and Facilities: Different services may be available in your community. These programs are available for those in need of constant support. You will find fun activities, therapy, food, and other health-related care options. For example, adult day centers offer relief for those with Alzheimer's by providing fun art or music programs. Here are some resources to learn more:

- Caring.com - https://www.caring.com/local/adult-day-care
- A Place for Mom - http://www.aplaceformom.com/respite-care

- ARCH National Respite Network - http://
archrespite.org/respitelocator

Overlap Services: When you want to be at home but need a break, use either unpaid or paid providers to provide temporary 'companion services' to give you a few hours of relief. This can be very helpful during the holidays.

On-the-Go: If you are traveling with your aging loved one but hope to find some time for yourself, utilize respite services at your destination.

Make Your Own: Not finding a solution you like? Try creating your own network of other caregivers (in similar situations) and create a sharing community where you can schedule time off with each other's support. This will create larger network to use as a resource.

Why Should I Use Respite Care?

Respite allows you – as the caregiver – to take some time off from caregiving duties. This break could be a few hours here and there to run errands, or a couple of weeks a year to take business trips or vacations. Although the idea is common among caregivers, many don't take advantage of it.

By engaging in respite care, you will be identifying either family members or paid caregivers to provide temporary care for your aging loved one. By doing so, you can:

- Spend time with other loved ones in your immediate family
- Get the things you need to get done, done
- Take time for yourself and RELAX!

Respite provides a much-needed break from the challenges

faced by a family caregiver. Make sure to plan in advance even if you are taking just a few hours. Remember to discuss the options with your loved one and make sure they are comfortable with this temporary change. Talk to them when you return and get their feedback.

You deserve a break – look into respite care now and plan for a break tomorrow.

How to Keep Your Loved One Physically Safe

THIRTY-FOUR

How to Perform Background Checks on Professional Caregivers

Before you hire any professional home caregivers to help your loved one, you should absolutely validate their work history through background checks. The term background check (or investigation) can mean a variety of things, such as hiring a firm to do the research, reviewing an agency's report, or conducting research yourself online.

Why Should I Do a Background Check?

Conducting a background check is done to ensure your loved one is in safe and capable hands. You must make sure that whoever is entering your home can be trusted to administer medicine, monitor the health and well-being of your loved one, and effectively manage any emergency situation. You will want someone who has validated work experience and no criminal history.

If you are using a home-caregiver firm to help you hire a caregiver, you should first ask them if they can conduct background checks, how often they do these checks, and request to review the final report.

Conducting Research on Your Own

You can start your research by doing a simple Google search of the potential candidate's name. Doing a search online will produce a lot of information that may not pertain to your candidate, so it will take time to weed through the findings. A helpful tip is to use keywords associated with the full name of the individual you are looking for, as well as using the advanced search functions. You can also search for the person's social media accounts and other public records. A caregiver may even have reviews online if they have been hired before through an online hiring network such as Care-Linx.com, Care.com, etc.

This free search may yield some insightful information that can help you make your decision. However, it may be difficult to find certain important details. In addition to conducting an online search, you should ask for the contact information of at least three previous clients whom you can contact as a reference.

Hiring an Accredited Firm

You can also use a full-service firm to run a background check for you. If you are not sure how to find a firm, there is a list available through the National Association of Professional Background Screeners (NAPBS). The NAPBS has 70 accredited firms listed that can perform small to extensive background checks for you. The fees can start around $50 – $80 and go up from there based on the type of search conducted.

You have the right to perform a background check if you so choose to. Use the information above to conduct your research using the method you feel is the best for you. Once you can validate the home caregiver's history, you should move forward with an offer. Take these steps now to protect your aging loved one.

THIRTY-FIVE

How to Identify and Prevent Elder Abuse

"My mom is in a memory care center. I feel at times she is being abused. They leave her wet. She has to be feed because she cannot eat on her own. They try once or twice to feed her, and then they are done trying. The caregiver that is supposed to give her her medication doesn't because she feels like it takes too much trouble. There is another elder in her area that yells all the time and wakes everyone up. The state is now involved because of short staff, medication control issues, and falls."

Did you know that 1 in 10 Americans aged 60+ have experienced some form of elder abuse? Although difficult to talk about, elder abuse is an important topic to understand and discuss in order to protect your aging loved ones from harm.

What is Elder Abuse?

According to the National Council on Aging (NCOA), elder abuse is really any form of mistreatment or a harmful act that results in injury, harm, or loss to an older person. This can be perpetrated by a person physically, emotionally, sexually, as well as through exploitation, neglect (which is more common than you may think), and abandonment.

Elder abuse is not just committed by criminals and scammers. Those perpetrating elder abuse can include family members, spouses, and staff members at nursing homes, assisted living, and other facilities, as well as those targeting older adults as easier targets for exploitation and abuse. Those looking to take advantage of your aging loved one may target them with internet scams, tax scams, telemarketing scams, or selling fraudulent products (i.e., anti-aging skincare).

Other abuses can occur both with malicious intent and without. For example, someone may be neglected on purpose to cause harm, or it could be unknown neglect due to poor communication and transparency.

Discussing Elder Abuse with Your Family

Identifying Elder Abuse

Now that you have a better understanding of elder abuse, you should discuss the potential warning signs with your entire family and caring village. The warning signs include:

- Physical abuse, neglect, or mistreatment: Bruises, broken bones, burn marks
- Emotional abuse: Unexplained withdrawal from normal activities, a sudden change in alertness, or unusual depression

- Financial abuse (exploitation): Sudden and extreme changes in financial situations
- Neglect (including self-neglect): Bedsores, unattended medical needs, poor hygiene, unusual weight loss
- Verbal or emotional abuse: Threats, or other uses of an imbalance of power and control by individuals

You should be actively looking out for elder abuse. Doing so will help all those involved to be able to identify it and quickly work to address it.

Preventing Elder Abuse

Openly discussing elder abuse with your family and aging loved one will help to proactively prevent and screen for potential abuse. Having open communication, which includes active listening, can help. If you do keep an open dialogue you should be focused on the following:

- Listen actively to your aging loved one for any signs of abuse
- Don't dismiss any warning signs, instead be proactive and transparent with all family members involved
- Engage in an open dialogue around your aging loved one's care if cared for at home or a care facility.
- Agree to pay attention and watch for changes in your aging family member's mood or appearance, to look for signs of abuse or neglect.
- Encourage your aging family member to be cautious in financial matters and to seek counsel before making financial decisions.

Another important way to prevent financial exploitation is by speaking with your family member about executing certain documents such as a will, living will, or durable power of attorney for health care and financial purposes.

If you suspect your loved one may be a victim of elder abuse – openly discuss your concerns with the person and encourage him or her to be open with you. Set your loved one's mind at ease and tell them that you are there to listen and assist in whatever way you can. If you have or suspect a real situation, you should immediately report it.

THIRTY-SIX

How to Prepare for a Weather Emergency

Weather emergencies can happen anywhere and at any time. Some parts of the U.S. are more accustomed to certain types of severe weather, but no one is completely safe – just consider snowstorms in Atlanta or hurricanes in New Jersey. To help you prepare for anything, make sure to know the weather risks in your area and take the following precautions.

"I find the best way to manage during bad weather is to stay prepared at all times, so I don't have to join the throngs of panic-stricken shoppers scavenging for the last quart of milk or the last package of batteries at the store. Refill meds well before they run out, keep the cars gassed up, Keep cell phones charged, keep the oil tank filled, have enough gas on hand for the generator. Plan as though you're going to be housebound and without power for a couple of days. And have some cash on hand. Even if you can get out and about, if the power is out, the ATMs won't work. Check battery stock and discard expired ones. Know where everything you might need is -- flashlights, outerwear, shovels, matches, candles, etc. Keep bottled water on hand if you're on a well."

Know the Weather Risks in Your Area

Begin by doing your own research into what types of hazardous weather typically affects where you live and when. This can include understanding your house's elevation, proximity to streams and rivers, the history of weather emergencies and other facts you can find both online and from your local government officials. The common types of weather-related emergencies can include:

- Tornadoes
- Floods
- Forest fires
- Severe thunderstorms and lightning
- Hurricanes
- Blizzards

12 Steps to Get Prepared Before Severe Weather Strikes

The National Safety Council recommends the following general precautions that apply to many disaster situations:

1. Create a family communication plan that includes where to meet in an emergency, how to reach each other by having all contact information and a plan to account for everyone after a disaster occurs
2. Have the communication essentials available, including a battery-powered radio to listen to local emergency broadcasts
3. Ensure you have a short-term back-up power source to charge your cell phones for emergency purposes

4. Have a back-up generator for longer periods of power outages (especially in locations with high or low temperatures)

5. Know who your local authorities are and follow them on social media for updates

6. Prepare and keep an emergency kit in your car and at least three days of food and water at home (Tip – have this in your house in advance of regular weather emergencies to avoid long lines even shortages at grocery stores)

7. Be sure to store all important documents – birth certificates, insurance policies, etc. – in a fire-proof safe or safety deposit box

8. Have several family members trained in first aid and CPR in case emergency responders are delayed

9. Know how to shut off your utilities, including pipes in the winter, electricity in flood and other potential emergencies situations

10. Know your local evacuation routes

11. Keep your car with a full tank of gas if possible (no less than half of a tank)

12. Have materials to board up your windows on hand, if necessary

Remember to keep these tips in mind as you prepare before severe weather strikes. In addition, always follow the directions from your local authorities. Get your family organized and be prepared as much as possible.

THIRTY-SEVEN

What You Need in a Home First-Aid Kit

In an emergency, having what you need when you need it can prevent further injury and infection. It is especially important to have first-aid supplies for older adults since they are more susceptible to injury and infection and take longer to recover. Whether you have a home first-aid kit, or still need to get one, review the suggested tips and tricks below to make sure you have what you need.

What Should Be in a Home First-Aid Kit?

Before filling up your home first-aid kit, you will want to consider the following:

- Use a kit that has wheels as it may become heavy with supplies
- Label your kit with your contact information
- Place your kit in an easily accessible location

A pre-made first-aid kit can be purchased at many locations (i.e., CVS, Walgreens, The American Red Cross) or you can build your own. Either way, these are the items that your first-aid kit should contain:

- Band-Aids, gauze, tape, ace bandages, cotton balls, and cotton swabs
- Tweezers, scissors, safety pins, and needles
- Plastic bags for trash and disposable items
- Antiseptic ointment and wipes, antibiotics, hand sanitizer, lotion
- Gloves, a thermometer, eye goggles
- Cold pack, thermal patches, blanket
- List of medication(s) along with dosage and schedule
- Flashlight and extra batteries
- Phone numbers of emergency contacts, doctors, pharmacy, poison control
- Blood pressure monitor (if applicable)
- Pain reliever, fever reducer, antihistamine, anti-diarrheal

The list above will not cover every type of emergency but should help in many situations. You should keep the kit somewhere easily accessible. Having a kit in the car will also give you comfort when you are on the road. Don't hesitate to add to this list and include items that are particularly important for you and your aging loved one. Remember to review your kit every six months to check for expired medicine and batteries and to replace or add anything new. Get yourself prepared today for the unexpected tomorrow.

THIRTY-EIGHT

Important Vaccinations for Aging Adults

Vaccines can save lives, prevent serious illness, and keep you healthy. Unfortunately, according to the Center for Disease Control (CDC), one in three seniors each year skips the flu vaccine and between 71% and 85% of seasonal flu-related deaths have occurred in people 65 years and older. If you are aging adult, or provide care for an aging adult, it's important to make sure you and your loved one are up to date with vaccinations, especially during National Immunization Awareness Month (NIAM).

Recommended Vaccinations for Older Adults

The flu vaccine is just one of several that older adults should receive. For adults aged 60+, the following vaccines are recommended:

- Flu Vaccine: Influenza (Flu)
- Zoster Vaccine: Shingles (Herpes Zoster)
- Td (tetanus, diphtheria) and Tdap (tetanus, diphtheria, and pertussis) vaccines: Diphtheria; Tetanus; Pertussis (Whooping Cough)

- Pneumococcal Vaccine: Pneumococcal disease (Pneumonia)

There is a good chance you have not received all of the vaccines needed, and there is no need to panic. We often don't realize what vaccines we need (especially beyond the flu vaccine, which is highly marketed). Remember that vaccines are safe and are intended to keep you healthy. You can get your vaccine at your doctor's office, pharmacy, and other community health centers.

Other items that will impact what vaccines you may need include travel plans, family history, age, allergies, chronic illnesses, timing with other vaccines, and more. The CDC has created a quick quiz to find out what vaccines you may need, and you can find the link in our Appendix section at the end of this book. Once you complete the quiz, take the list with you to your doctor and discuss your results to find out which vaccines are recommended for you based on your specific health status, age, and lifestyle.

Will Medicare Pay for Your Vaccine?

In most cases, Medicare Part B will pay for the following vaccines:

- Influenza (flu) vaccine
- Pneumococcal vaccines
- Hepatitis B vaccines for persons at increased risk of hepatitis

In addition, Medicare Part D or Medicare Advantage Plan Part C may also have partial or full coverage for other vaccines, including:

- Shingles vaccine
- MMR vaccine
- Td and Tdap vaccines
- Hepatitis A

Remember that we receive many vaccines as a child but typically don't think about continuing to get them as we age. You need to be proactive and discuss what vaccines you may need with your doctor. So, join millions of others during National Immunization Awareness Month and get vaccinated to protect your health and well-being.

THIRTY-NINE

Does My Loved One Need a Home Alert System?

Your loved ones' well-being is important to you, and you want to look out for their health and safety. As they age, their likelihood of falling and the susceptibility to injury increases. While the initial impact of a fall may be minimal, having a Home Alert System can be reassuring in the case of an emergency. Not only will this protection help to keep your loved ones safe, but it can also give you peace-of-mind.

A Home Alert system (also called a Personal Emergency Response System, Medical Alert or Medical Emergency Response System) will instantly contact a response team with 24/7 monitoring. Some examples include Bay Alarm Medical, Medical Guardian, ADT, and more.

Why Are Home Alert Systems Important?

In 2014, emergency departments treated 2.8 million nonfatal falls among older adults, and more than 800,000 of these patients were hospitalized. One out of three older adults (65 and older) falls each year. That number does not immediately equal devastating injuries to those individuals, but some of the impacts can include, according to the CDC:

- Twenty to thirty percent of people who fall suffer moderate to severe injuries such as lacerations, hip fractures, and head traumas. These injuries can make it hard to get around or live independently and increase the risk of early death.
- Falls are the most common cause of traumatic brain injuries (TBI).
- About one-half of fatal falls among older adults are due to TBI.
- Most fractures among older adults are caused by falls. The most common are fractures of the spine, hip, forearm, leg, ankle, pelvis, upper arm, and hand.
- Many people who fall, even if they are not injured, develop a fear of falling. This fear may cause them to limit their activities, which leads to reduced mobility and loss of physical fitness, and in turn, increases their actual risk of falling.

How to Choose a Home Alert System

The following are useful evaluative metrics to review when shopping for a Home Alert System:

- **Price** (flat fee or monthly) – consider how you will have to pay for the system and who will be paying the bill (you or your loved one).
- **Ease of Use** – consider how complicated the system is and how quickly you can learn to use it.
- **Source of Power** (battery or rechargeable) – consider if you have to recharge the system and where you will recharge it. If battery-powered, keep a supply of batteries on hand.

- **Connectivity** – consider how the system connects with local authorities and if there are any potential obstructions within your home.
- **Size** – consider the size and weight of the device.
- **Comfort** – consider if your loved one is comfortable carrying the device around.

A home alert system is a great way to prevent injury or mitigate any emergency situations. Start researching today and consider the metrics above when reviewing home alert systems. For more information, check out The Top Ten Home Alert Systems.

FORTY

The Top 10 Home Alert Systems

Home alert systems allow users to contact emergency services in the event of a fall or other emergency. If you recently determined that your aging loved one needs a home alert system, here is the Consumers Advocate's list of the Top 10 best medical alert products for 2017:

Medical Guardian: Medical Guardian's mission is to provide an affordable and reliable medical alert service to all those who wish to live an independent life, regardless of their limitations. Whether customers are looking to remain safe in a medical emergency (such as a seizure, stroke, or heart attack), have limited mobility, are at risk of falling as they age, or are afraid to live alone because of home invasions or fires, Medical Guardian guarantees that they will be there to protect them.

Bay Alarm Medical: Bay Alarm Medical provides consultation, technical support, and customer service from their headquarters in California. They keep 24/7 medical monitoring completely separate from their day-to-day business operations to ensure that all calls are rapidly responded to. In the case of a medical emergency, pushing the help button quickly connects your loved one to a professionally-trained operator.

MobileHelp: MobileHelp isn't the least expensive option, but they're certainly among the best. The company provides a reliable GPS-enabled medical alert system that helps protect loved ones at home and away from home. MobileHelp offers a host of peripheral features, including automatic fall detection and location tracking.

GreatCall: GreatCall is committed to supporting the needs of aging Americans and the approximately 42 million family members who care for them with innovative products and services that keep families connected while preserving independence.

Medical Alert: Connect America, Medical Alert, and/or Alarm Company specializes in Personal Emergency Response Services (PERS). Connect America is a nationwide company founded by Kenneth Gross, with its corporate headquarters in Broomall, Pennsylvania. Connect America's core business is providing personal emergency monitoring and home alarm services nationwide to older adults with medical ailments or conditions, who wish to live at home.

Philips Lifeline: Philips Lifeline is a Massachusetts-based medical alert provider. Originally Lifeline Solutions, the company was acquired by Philips in 2006. With both wireless and landline options, this company's medical alerts can be used at home or on the go. Features include auto alert and quick dialing, and their fall detection software boasts a 95% success rate.

LifeStation: LifeStation has been instrumental in providing a safety net for those faced with the potential of requiring immediate medical assistance. The LifeStation medical monitoring system has been designed by industry veterans who have one goal in mind — secured independence.

ADT: When an alarm signal is received from the personal emergency response system, you can count on this professional monitoring system to deliver a fast response to both you and the appropriate response agency.

Medical Care Alert: Medical Care Alert is a company that provides medical alert services for seniors. It has a variety of medical alert plans and equipment designed to notify medical professionals about any emergency.

LifeFone: LifeFone has been an innovator in providing security and peace of mind to thousands of people throughout the U.S. since 1976. Utilizing the latest information technology and their continued commitment to "personal" response, Life-Fone is at the forefront of the healthcare communications industry.

Explore each of the products listed above to find the one that best meets your aging loved one's needs. You can also discuss these options with your healthcare provider to get their recommendation. Remember that finding the right product can give you peace of mind and protect your loved one.

FORTY-ONE

Does My Loved One Need a Bed Rail?

Getting in and out of a bed can often be quite difficult for an older adult due to common health problems such as decreased strength and pain from movement. Bed rails can make this task safer and easier.

What Are Bed Rails?

Bed rails are railings that go along the side of a bed and connect to both the headboard and footboard, preventing a person lying on the bed from rolling out easily. Bed rails may take on various titles such as bed side rails, half rails, safety rails, bed handles, assist bars, hospital bed rails, and adult portable bed rails.

When Should You Use a Bed Rail?

A bed rail should be used to:

- Reduce the risk of falling from the bed since an injury from falling can have serious health risks including broken bones, internal damage, etc.

- Help your parent reposition in the bed on his or her own.
- Help your parent get in and out of bed on his or her own.
- In general, a bed rail should be used when someone has poor strength, decreased flexibility, poor endurance, and general difficulty moving around.

A bed rail should not be used:

- As a restraint to keep your parent in a bed even if they have a physical or mental need. It is dangerous without proper supervision. This can potentially cause suffocation, injury, neglect, and/or entrapment.
- Without proper installment, so that it does not cause injury or harm to your parent.

The **overall advantages of using bed rails (when appropriate) include:**

- increasing your parent's safety
- preventing falls
- promoting independence.

Overall, a bed rail will give your parent the autonomy and freedom to move in and out of his or her bed at will without assistance (unless needed). The bed rail can provide comfort and confidence. If you think you should purchase a bed rail for your parent, then be sure to keep reading to find out how to find the best bed rail for your aging parent.

FORTY-TWO

How to Select the Best Bed Rails

A simple task, such as getting in and out of bed, can be extremely difficult for some older adults. If you have a parent that is having difficulty getting into or out of bed, repositioning in bed, or is at risk of falling or rolling out of bed, then a bed rail may be the right answer. Once you've decided it's time to purchase a bed rail, it's time to do some research to find out the bed rail that will be the best for you or your loved one.

How to Select the Best Bed Rail for Your Needs

ParentGiving.com provides an easily searchable environment for bed rail products and offers the following questionnaire to identify which bed rail is right for your parent:

- What kind of bed will the rail be used on? Is there a box spring and mattress? Is it an adjustable bed? Is it a hospital bed? What size is the bed?
- Do they want the rail to be one-sided or two?
- Will the rail be used as an assist to help them get in

and out of bed, or is it to keep them in bed during the night? (or both?)

- Is there a caregiver to raise and lower the rail, or will the patient need to do that him or herself? Before purchasing a bedrail for use in a facility, it is important to contact the facility and determine what can and cannot be installed.
- If a loved one suffers from dementia and is quite active, will they be confused and try to climb over the rails? Rather than protecting the patient, this could actually harm them more.

After doing your research, the next step is to select the right bed rail. You will also want to consider price points before making the final purchase. In general, bed rails cost between $50 to $150 depending on the design. Make sure you shop around to compare prices across stores.

What to Do After Choosing a Bed Rail

The Consumer Protection Safety Commission provides the following checklist to follow after choosing a bed rail:

- Check with the manufacturer to make sure the bed rails are compatible with the mattress and bed frame. These are not one-size-fits-all products.
- Select and place bed rails in a way that discourages climbing over the rails to get in and out of bed, which can lead to falling over the rails.
- Install bed rails using the manufacturer's instructions to ensure a proper fit.
- Check bed rails regularly and readjust as needed to make sure they are installed correctly. Rails can shift or loosen over time, creating dangerous gaps.
- Check for recalled bed rails or handles. (You can do

this right on the Consumer Protection Safety
Commission website.)

Each bed rail will have its own instructions on how to install.
Some bed rails are secured with straps and clips, others are
attached to the metal bed frame, and others are fitted and
weighted down by the mattress. Make sure to read the instructions carefully and secure the bed rail properly to ensure your
parent's safety and wellbeing.

FORTY-THREE

The Top 10 Stair Lift Companies

If your parent has mobility issues and requires the assistance of a walking cane, walker, or wheelchair, then you may also want to consider installing a stairlift in either your home (if they currently reside with you) or in their home.

Stairlifts (also known as chair lifts) allow users to sit comfortably in a seat that takes them up the steps using the stairs' railing as a track. According to Consumers Advocate, the top ten stairlift companies are Harmar, AmeriGlide, Improvement Center, Handicare, Stannah, 101 Mobility, Ascent, Acorn, Bruno, and EHLS. Learn more about each of these companies and how stairlifts work below.

The Top 10 Stair Lift Companies

Harmar

Harmar has the largest variety of wheelchair, scooter, and power stairlifts and offers innovative solutions to enhance home accessibility for the mobility-challenged. Harmar provides people with a way to gain more freedom to go where they want, when they want. Harmar offers ergonomically designed seats and a 2-year warranty on standard lifts.

AmeriGlide

AmeriGlide offers nationwide measuring and installation. In addition, you have the option to do it yourself, which could potentially save hundreds of dollars. The price for this product starts at $1,540. It has a weight capacity of up to 500 lbs and comes with servicing and repair options.

Improvement Center

Improvement Center helps consumers easily connect with local stairlift providers and installers by simply filling up an online form and submitting their zip code. After submitting the information, consumers are provided with several quotes from different stairlift contractors without an obligation to purchase.

Handicare

Handicare is committed to making everyday life easier for disabled and elderly people and to empowering them to live an active life – on their terms. At the same time, they want to support those who assist them. This is why they provide well-designed solutions that help increase independence and are easy and safe to use for both healthcare professionals and family members.

Stannah

Stannah is recognized around the world as the company that brings freedom, independence, and a strong sense of safety back to anyone who has difficulty overcoming the challenges posed by the stairs in their home. The Stannah stairlift is fully customizable, and the company will do a free assessment with no obligation to purchase. Stannah stairlifts are offered by more than 200 dealers nationwide.

101 Mobility

101 Mobility provides a variety of stairlifts and mobility solutions from its personally manufactured equipment and known brands nationwide. The company offers products such as auto lifts, incline platform lifts, vertical platform lifts, stairlifts, scooters, wheelchair ramp maintenance, and limited use elevators.

Ascent Stair Lifts

Ascent Stair Lifts was established in 2008, after many years of experience in the accessibility industry. In the beginning, Ascent had the simple yet ambitious idea of providing the best mobility products and services at affordable prices. The goal of Ascent has always been to help customers feel safe in their homes and regain the confidence and independence that is so deserved by all.

Acorn Stair Lifts

Acorn Stair Lifts is an international, family-owned company that employs thousands worldwide. Their core business is the manufacture, sale, and service of stairlifts. Acorn prides itself with creating the most contemporary design, using the latest innovations, and manufacturing top-quality components. Acorn Stair Lifts has pioneered the use of direct current (DC) batteries, the FastTrack system, and Smart-Level technology.

Bruno

Bruno is an ISO certified manufacturer that offers independent lifestyle solutions to mobility-challenged individuals and elders. The company provides products with patented swivel technology such as mobility device lifts for vehicles, stairlifts, valet signature seating, and vertical platform lifts. Bruno offers a range of budget-wise stairlifts that helps seniors and mobility-challenged individuals restore safety and gain peace of mind in their own homes.

EHLS, a Lifeway Mobility Company

EHLS, a Lifeway Mobility Company, is a local, family-run stairlift company that helps those with limited mobility regain their independence and stay safe in their homes. They are a Bruno Diamond Stair Lift Dealer and have been serving the greater Chicago area, including northwest Indiana and southeast Wisconsin since 1991. Some of the other products offered by EHLS are ramps, wheelchair lifts, bathroom modifications, and home elevators. Lifeway Mobility, proudly provides a wide variety of accessible solutions to those living in CT, IN, IL, MA, MN, & RI.

Additional Information

There are two basic types of stairlifts that are sold today: straight and curved. The best lifts include features that maximize comfort, are easy to use, and aesthetically pleasing. The type you need depends upon the design of your staircase. Keep in mind that prices for a simple stairlift for straight stairs often range between $2000 to $4000, but for more elaborate stairways and chairs, the price can be as much as $15,000 (or even more, in some cases).

When purchasing a stairlift, make sure you do your research and discuss your options with a physician. There is a great company called the Buyer Zone that provides stairlift buyer assistance for families who might not be sure of the best lift for their home. You can answer a few questions about your home or office at Caring Village, and the Buyer Zone will connect you with local professionals to help you with your installation.

FORTY-FOUR

What Are the Top 10 Products to Track My Elderly Loved One's Location?

"Mom has had Alzheimer's for over ten years without declining below the first stage. Recently, she had two incidents that concern me. First, she woke up thinking she was on a boat. She yelled out the front door for help, but she stayed in the house because it was "too cold to swim." I found out after she called 9-1-1 and the sheriff called me. The second incident she left the house (a double-wide in my back yard) around 2 am and returned after a few minutes. If she hadn't returned, I would not have known until the next morning. I would not want her out in her PJs for several hours on a cold winter night."

The number of people living with dementia and Alzheimer's Disease is expected to rise to 75.6 million by 2030, and 135.5 million by 2050 (source)[2]. Dementia and other similar conditions often cause older adults to become disoriented or lost in both familiar and unfamiliar places.

The use of GPS technology like that offered by AngelSense, Pocketfinder, iTraq, Trax, Spy Tec, Yepzon, SPOT, GPS SmartSole, Trackimo and Medical Guardian can bring your aging loved one safely home and provide greater peace of mind for caregivers and family members. Below is our list of the top 10 GPS products for tracking your aging loved one's location based on reviews from several tech industry blogs, customer reviews, and ratings.

Top 10 Products to Track my Elderly Parents Location

AngelSense Elderly GPS Tracker and App
The AngelSense GPS Tracker is a unique offering that combines a GPS tracker and mobile app with a monthly service plan that includes unlimited notifications, full-day location updates, late departure warnings, email alerts, and real-time technical support. AngelSense initially entered the market as a service to track children and those with special needs (such as autism) and then eventually expanded into the elderly tracking space. This solution is perfect for individuals with Dementia, Alzheimer's Disease, and other memory problems as it helps prevent wandering and mistreatment while promoting independence and reducing family caregiver stress and anxiety. The AngelCall feature also allows families to talk to their elderly loved one directly without the need for them to "pick-up" the device. Angelsense offers three pricing plans and provides free onboarding support by phone.

PocketFinder
The latest PocketFinder Trackers launched in January 2017. The newer model utilizes all three location technologies, GPS,

Cell ID, and Google Wi-Fi touch, for accurate outdoor and indoor locating. It also has an SOS button. Receive $30 off Personal or Vehicle trackers with discount code: CARING30

iTraq

iTraq determines its position using WiFi triangulation (for indoor tracking) as well as GPS and cellular tower triangulation that allows iTraq to be located anywhere in the world where cellular service exists. There's also fall detection, scheduled reporting, and geofencing capabilities. In some configurations, battery life can also last up to four months.

Trax

Trax is the smallest and lightest real-time tracker on the market, combining GPS and GLONASS for increased precision. Single or multiple trackers can be monitored via easy-to-use smartphone (iOS/Android) and desktop web apps. Trax boasts an array of features including geofence security, proximity and speed alerts, and an Augmented Reality fast-find feature. Trax is small in size but big on technology and fits easily into a pocket or bag.

Spy Tec Mini GPS Tracker

The Spy Tec STI_GL300 Mini Portable Real Time GPS Tracker is a good match for seniors because it ensures unsurpassed accuracy and provides real-time location tracking. Powered by proprietary tracking software and the cutting-edge GL-300 real-time GPS tracking device, Spy Tec is an industry leader in addressing consumer and enterprise GPS tracking needs. On Amazon, this product received a 4.5 (out of 5) rating with 1,533 reviews to date.

Yepzon One Personal GPS Locator

The Yepzon GPS Locator tracks the location of your loved one every 10 seconds. It can work with any mobile device and the battery life is suitable to last several weeks (to even months) depending on how often you need to use it. On Amazon, this product received a 4 (out of 5) rating with more than 250 comments and reviews.

SPOT 3 Satellite GPS Messenger

SPOT Gen3 gives aging adults a critical, life-saving line of communication when they travel beyond the boundaries of cell service. The latest generation of award-winning SPOT devices, SPOT Gen3 lets family and friends know their loved one is okay, or if the worst should happen, sends emergency responders their GPS location – all with the push of a button.

GPS SmartSole

The GPS SmartSole provides peace of mind for family members and those caring for the millions of people suffering from memory impairment and wandering which can be caused by Alzheimer's, Dementia, Autism, Traumatic Brain Injury, or other cognitive memory disability. The patented GPS enabled "Smart" insoles fit easily into most adult shoes and let you monitor the whereabouts of loved ones who may tend to wander or be at risk of becoming disoriented and lost. You can track their location through any smartphone, tablet, or web browser, set up text and e-mail alerts if they leave or enter defined areas on a map. This product received a 3.9 (out of 5) star review on Amazon.

Trackimo

Trackimo has a comprehensive GPS tracker offering to include uses for vehicles, drones, pets, children and the elderly. Their primary device is currently the smallest on the market coming in at less than 1.5 ounces. Trackimo leverages smart alerts by SMS or email that can automatically message family members when their loved one leaves the "safe zone." They also boast about a battery life of up to 96 hours, which is quite impressive with the small size of the device. As of November of 2018, they are offering free GPS service for the first year before you transition into a $5 per month fee, which is the lowest fee we are aware of. Although their primary device is the 3G Tracker, their other devices such as travel trackers, watches and pet devices all have the same functionality in different form factors and can be reviewed at their online store.

Medical Guardian

Medical Guardian provides numerous options for families and seniors such as GPS trackers, medical alert devices, in-home devices and personal emergency response systems. Their offerings also include fall detection and a 24/7 monitoring service that provides a comprehensive security offering. Their newest product, the Freedom Guardian, resembles modern-day smartwatches which is much more discrete than other similar offerings but still easy to operate. Medical Guardian's devices are consistently ranked highly in numerous online review sources such as Consumers Advocate, Reviews.com, Medical Alert Comparisons and others.

Before purchasing a GPS tracking device, make sure to receive permission from your aging loved one. Although GPS tracking does not necessarily equal better care, as it cannot stop someone from getting lost, if worn or in possession of the person lost, they can provide peace of mind to concerned family members. Research the products above to find the right device or app for you or your loved one.

How to Keep Your Loved One Safe Financially

FORTY-FIVE

How to Protect Those with Alzheimer's and Dementia from Financial Abuse

"My mother-in-law and I have Power of Attorney of her 98-year old mother. One of her granddaughters stole money from her in the past and has now taken her to a lawyer and made out a new will. Grandma has Alzheimer's and has had it for a few years, and the past, year she has really gotten bad. Grandma is not of her right mind to be signing anything! "

Every year seniors lose up to $36.5 billion from various types of financial abuse and exploitation. This is a serious matter and one that deserves attention, particularly for those diagnosed with Alzheimer's and/or Dementia. These cognitive conditions make older adults even more susceptible to scammers and criminals. In a previous section of this book, we described how to identify and prevent elderly abuse by acknowledging that anyone can perpetrate this type of abuse (including strangers, telemarketers, and even family and friends). There is no fail-proof way to stop elder financial abuse, but there are a few things you can do right now to protect your aging parent with dementia or Alzheimer's. We've outlined seven of these steps below.

7 Steps to Prevent Financial Abuse

1. Put in place a financial power of attorney immediately. By making yourself your aging parent's power of attorney, you ensure that a legal document is in place based on state law that empowers a succession of individuals (you) to make financial decisions and handle administrative affairs on behalf of your parent.

2. Create a profile of all names, contact information, and other important data points of the banking, financial, and other legal institutions/professionals your parent is engaged with.

3. Add your name to all of your parents' bank and financial accounts. Request that a duplicate copy of each monthly statement is also delivered to you. This will enable a second pair of eyes to review each statement and monitor for any irregular activity.

4. Hire a licensed professional fiduciary agent who can take over the responsibility of paying bills and managing assets. Make a provision in the Power of Attorney to have a third party review the appointed person's actions.

5. Set up automatic bill pay and direct deposits. This doesn't just save time; it keeps your loved one away from bill paying, which can prevent mistakes and won't create easy opportunities for scammers.

6. Do your research on those providing care for your aging parent. Conduct background checks on

caregivers or require a background investigation report of any hired from in-home care providers.

7. Keep a watchful eye out for any warning signs such as payments to individuals you are unfamiliar with; unpaid bills, irregular spending activity, transfer of funds, purchases of gift cards or other behavior you feel stands out. Immediately report anything that seems strange.

These are just a few ways to prevent abuse. If abuse does occur, you should report it to the bank and the authorities immediately. According to the American Bankers Association (ABA), "Financial institutions can play a key role in addressing elder financial exploitation due to the nature of the client relationship. Often, financial institutions are quick to suspect elder financial exploitation based on bank personnel familiarity with their elderly customers. The valuable role financial institutions can play in alerting appropriate authorities to suspected elder financial exploitation has received increased attention at the state level; this focus is consistent with an upward trend at the federal level in Suspicious Activity Reports (SARs) describing instances of suspected elder financial exploitation."

Although the banks may be able to identify irregular activity – the financial exploitation may occur in other ways as well. Having your name on your parents' bank accounts, ensuring you have installed power of attorney, and being included on financial statements will get you ahead of what many unfortunately experience.

FORTY-SIX

How to Protect Your Loved One from Telemarketing and Phone Scams

"A new scam is making the rounds where I live. A person will call up saying they are from the electric company and they will be turning off your electricity unless you pay your outstanding bill of $300."

How many times have you had to give out your phone number in the past two weeks? You try to protect it, but we use it everywhere. Now, put your 'what if' hat on and consider the following scenario: it is a quiet Saturday afternoon, and your mom gets a phone call gets a call telling her she has been selected as a winner for a special prize.

Instead of hanging up, she is intrigued. The caller asks for her home address and credit card number to make sure she is the correct winner, and she provides it. All of this happens in under a minute, and the caller says 'thank you' and says they will be in touch. This is a phone scam.

Scammers will try and sound and seem like normal sales representatives. It is your job to be on the lookout and educate your aging loved one on how to be prepared and prevent a telemarketing/phone scam from becoming a reality. These scams are real and can easily infiltrate your home. Use the recommendations below to be ready anytime for what could be a harmful scam.

How to Prevent a Telemarketing or Phone Scam from Becoming Reality

The best ways to prevent you or your loved one from becoming the target of a telemarketing scam is to take some preliminary preventative measures and to know how to identify the signs of a scam.

Know How to React to a Scam
If you encounter a phone scam, your best option is to hang-up, but you need to be ready for the call, so you are not caught off guard. You can protect yourself by:

Protecting Your Phone Number: Be restrictive on giving out your phone number as much as possible. It is hard these days when so many stores and offices require a phone number but remember that it's okay to ask why the company needs your number. If it is not required, don't provide it.

Not Giving into the Time Pressure: Scammers will often push to give them your private information quickly. If you are in doubt, then ask for more information from the caller or ask to call them back. You will be able to quickly assess the situation based on their response.

Not Paying for a Free Prize or Special Offer: Think

about it, why would you have to pay for a prize or special offer? Also, ask how you were selected for this prize and don't give out your private financial information.

Know What a Telemarketer/Phone Scam Sounds Like

Those calling to steal your information will often make the following requests:

You have been chosen for a specific offer that requires you to provide personal information (i.e., credit card information, social security numbers, etc.) in order to receive it.

You are a winner and "the prize is yours," if you can charge the shipping and handling on your credit card.

There is a great investment opportunity for you, and it is low risk, but you must get involved today.

You are asked to donate to a charity that you have never heard of, and you need to donate today (starting with a small sum of money).

Listen for these keywords and phrases if someone you don't know calls you. Typically, the caller will put a lot of pressure on you to act quickly and to not to ask anyone else for his or her opinion.

You need to remember that scams can come in many different ways. The suggestions and tips above are only common cases and ways to prevent falling for a scam. Use common sense when talking with anyone on the phone if you're asked to provide personal, financial information.

FORTY-SEVEN

How to Protect Your Aging Loved Ones from Tax Scams

"My 89-year-old mom, who is of sound mind, has lost most of her money to a scam. She refuses to believe it and thinks that with "one last payment," she will get her money back. She doesn't believe my sister and me when we tell her this is a scam and show her stories about the scammer. How can we maintain her dignity and privacy in this moment yet extract her from this brainwashing?"

A new year, a new tax scam. Each tax season there are scammers lurking on the internet, over the phone, and sometimes even in-person. It is unfortunate, but if you have aging parents or loved ones, it is important that you are aware of tax scams targeting the elderly.

Criminals are finding new and creative ways to scam your loved ones out of their money online, on the phone, in-person, and by mail. It's especially important to be aware of this during tax season. You can help protect your loved ones from tax scams by knowing what the IRS will never do and which types of scams to look out for.

Common Tax Scams to Watch For

Phone Scams: Criminals may call your parents and impersonate an IRS agent claiming to need personal information such as a social security number, date-of-birth, etc. The fake caller may suggest that not disclosing this information will result in arrest or other charges.

Phishing Emails: Emails are an easy way for scammers to send phony messages requesting your parent provide personal information, banking information, or re-file their taxes. In many cases, the email will look and feel like a real IRS request, and the link will take you to a 'look-a-like' website.

These scams can often look like:

- Requesting fake tax payments – the IRS will never call for immediate payment, especially through prepaid debit cards or other forms of money transfers.
- The Federal Student Tax – this is a common one that says the payment is overdue and the authorities will be called if it goes unpaid. There is no such law, and the IRS would not do that.
- Verifying tax return information over the phone – this is how criminals get your personal information by asking for your private information.
- Promises of big refunds – phone calls or emails about

tax refunds are scams hoping to reel you in with the idea of extra cash.

What the IRS Will Never Do

It is a sure bet that the IRS will never do the following:

- Call you directly and require payment over the phone, text message, email, or by social media. The IRS will mail you a letter directly.
- Prevent you from appealing or questioning the amount of taxes you may owe. The IRS will allow for appeals and payment plans to be set up depending on the situation.
- Expect or require you to use only one method of payment to pay your taxes (i.e., your checking account). The IRS will allow for multiple types of payment.
- Request your credit card, debit card, or your checking account number over the phone. The IRS has many other options to receive this information (i.e., online or via mail).
- Suggest the police will arrest you for not paying your taxes in full. The IRS will send explicit information to your home regarding penalties of not paying your taxes.

FORTY-EIGHT

How to Protect Your Loved Ones from Internet Scams

"My 85-year-old father has been traumatized by the sudden death of my younger brother so much so that he has been highly susceptible to internet scams which in previous years, he would've laughed at. He has lost upwards of $30,000 and possibly more in this past year alone to various scams. I did convince him to go to the FBI, and we filed an IC3 report, but so far nothing has been done (but it was less than two weeks ago; I know they are back-logged). He is still insisting that these "accounts" are real despite the fact that I keep telling him that the only money existing in these scenarios is the money he is putting OUT."

To protect your loved ones, you should:

- Instruct them to never give financial or personal information by phone, email, text, or social media to an unsolicited message. Contact the IRS directly.

- Prevent potential robocalls by contacting the phone provider and have them block any robocall numbers.
- Remain skeptical if you receive IRS emails or phone calls. When in doubt, contact the IRS to confirm the request.
- Do not open attachments or click on links in emails sent from the IRS.

When it comes to tax scams, the best way to protect your loved ones is to remain vigilant. If you or a loved one does get caught in an IRS scam, contact the IRS and authorities immediately.

How to Protect Your Loved One from Internet Scams

Imagine going online and seeing a link to win a free cruise. The link, website, and entry form look and feel legitimate. The form asks you for your name, address, and contact information, which is a common request and one we may be comfortable providing. Then the site asks for a credit card in order to enter your name. What should be your next action? This is an internet scam and just one of many different ways criminals are infiltrating you and your loved one's lives.

It can be difficult to differentiate between a legitimate website and a fake one, but there are several steps you can take to protect yourself from Internet scams. Anyone can be a victim of an internet scam, but older adults are common targets because they may not be as confident or as knowledgeable as those who grew up with the internet. Use the suggested tips below to educate and protect you and your loved one from internet scams.

4 Tips to Protect Against Internet Scams

1. **Update the computer's anti-virus and security software.** Take the time to update your loved one's computer protection software. There are many programs out there, so take your time researching the best product (if you don't already have one). This will help to prevent viruses from stealing any private information. Remember, only download programs from websites you know and trust.

2. **When making online purchases look for the padlock.** When entering your credit card information to make purchases, only do so through a secure network. This is commonly identified by the padlock symbol in the web browser followed by https://. If you don't see this symbol, think twice about entering in your information and research the company to make sure it is real.

3. **Avoid online entry forms that ask for your information.** Criminals will use what looks like a contest or free giveaway entry forms to draw in potential victims. You should only provide your credit card or bank account number if you are actually purchasing something from a company that you trust.

4. **Be on the lookout for unsolicited emails.** Don't open or respond to the email that requests you to send money immediately to someone you may or may not know. No matter how convincing the email may appear, it is a fake and is pulling at your emotions to help. Delete these emails immediately and mark the sender as spam or junk.

Remember, the best way to protect you or your loved one from internet scams is to remain vigilant. You can help your loved one by staying involved. Talk to them about internet scams and review the tips above as ways to prevent them.

Managing Medical Issues

FORTY-NINE

How to Get the Most Out of Your Doctor's Visits

Have you ever left a doctor's appointment feeling confused, wondering what to do next? Like many of us, the fact that you may not have gone to the appointment prepared, nor been completely honest with your physician or caregiver, may have resulted in a less than stellar experience for all parties. To help you get the most out of your next doctor's appointment, we've drafted some easy steps for you to follow in preparation for and during your visit.

Preparing for Your Doctor's Visits

Before your next appointment, consider taking just a few moments out of your day to prepare for it in advance. This preparation will allow you to make the best use of the often limited time you have with your doctor.

What you should do before visiting the doctor:

1. Write your questions down beforehand

2. Drink plenty of water before a physical to ensure you're hydrated

3. Eat as you normally would before a checkup

Also, keep in mind what you should not do before visiting the doctor:

1. Don't eat a high-fat meal before getting blood drawn

2. Don't drink coffee before a blood pressure test

3. Don't take cold medicine before a visit (if possible)

4. Don't drink alcohol before a cholesterol test

Now that you know how to prepare physically for your appointment, follow the list of 5 steps below to really get the most from your visit.

5 Easy Ways to Get the Most Out of Your Doctor Visits

Share Your Symptoms

Think about this beforehand. Consider what has been causing your pain or discomfort. Keep notes before the meeting in reference to frequency, level of pain, areas of discomfort, and other important facts. Bring the notes to your visit and be open to our doctor's question. They are asking for more information to help you. And you being open and honest about your experiences will help your doctor give you the best treatment.

Ask Questions

Prepare a list of questions beforehand as it relates to your visit. Bring those questions with you or email them to your doctor in advance if there are any specific items that may require research on their part. When at the appointment, go through your list and make sure your questions are answered or at least asked. If new questions come up, write them down or ask right there in the moment. If you have a friend or loved one with you, they can take notes for you.

Bring a Friend or Loved One

Having someone with you can be valuable in a few ways: as a companion, someone to transport you, someone to be available for difficult conversations, a note-taker and much more. Make sure you are comfortable with whoever is there being a part of private conversations. The more they are involved, the more likely they'll be able to help you after the visit as well.

Bring Your Medication(s)

Depending on the visit, you may need to share all of the medications you are currently taking. And depending on the size of the list you can either bring a written list or simply bring the medications themselves. If your visit relates to how you feel when taking a specific medication – you should bring that specific one (and note any others you take at the same time). Also, be mindful of referencing brand names versus generic names when referring to the specific medication you take.

Recap Before You Leave

Don't leave the visit with questions! Summarize your understanding of next steps at the end and ask the doctor to confirm you are correct. This recap will ensure that you leave with a clear sense of what to do next and reduce anxiety around next steps. Be sure to schedule a follow-up appointment if necessary before you leave.

Our Making the Most of Your Doctor's Appointment Checklist at https://www.caringvillage.com/checklists/doctors-visit/ will get you organized, help you feel confident and prepare you with important questions and information to consider. Use it before and after your next visit!

FIFTY

9 Tips for Managing Your Medications

"My mother was recently diagnosed with Alzheimer's. She's still living at home and is able to manage most of her own life. I found out, yesterday, that she has been forgetting to take her medications despite the daily organizer my sister and I have for her. I get the "oh, that's right," or "oh, yeah, I need a refill" when I bring it up, but the fact of the matter is that she didn't remember ever having them prescribed to her in the first place. My sister and I are trying to keep her as independent as possible for as long as possible, but she obviously needs a repetitive reminder for the medication issue."

By now, you understand why medication management is particularly important for aging adults. If you take multiple medications on a regular schedule, follow these helpful tips provided by NIH Senior Health to assist you in managing your prescriptions:

• **Keep a checklist** of the medications you currently take including the name, time you take them, how long you have taken them, and then continue to add to the list if and when new prescriptions are added. You can also you the free Caring Village app to store your medications.

• **Review your medicinal record** when you meet with your doctor. Keep a detailed list of the medicines you use and bring your checklist as a reference.

• **Ask your pharmacist to provide your medicine in large, easy-to-open containers with large-print labels.** Always keep your medicine in the original container unless using a daily pill box that allows you to put the appropriate pills in each day. Don't take a pill if you are not confident it is in the right pill bottle. Also, make sure the pill bottles are properly labeled and, if necessary, color code, or number them.

• **To determine how a medication should be stored,** consult with your doctor on location, temperature, and other requirements for medication storage.

• **Don't stop taking a prescription drug unless your doctor says it's okay**. Always continue through the prescription even if you are feeling better. Consult with your doctor before making any changes in your medication.

• **Get prescriptions refilled early enough so you won't run out of medicines.** Keep on top of your refill dates and expirations.

• **Keep all medicines out of sight and reach of children and away from pets.** Always keep your medication in a secure place that both children and pets cannot reach or access.

• **Purchase a medication management tool.** There are many medication management tools on the market today, such as pill dispensers, automatic reminders, and electronic medicine caps.

• **Download a Medication Management Mobile App.** Keep track of your medication, scheduling, and other specific needs via mobile apps on your phone or tablet.

Don't just follow one of the tips above but explore all of them. Managing your medications properly can mean the difference of time, health, and overall well-being. Always ask questions when you are unsure about your medication and, most importantly, keep track of what you are taking daily. This will aid in your recovery and keep you on target.

FIFTY-ONE

The Best Tools for Medication Management

If you have multiple errands to run on a Saturday, what would you do? Most likely, you would create a list in order of priority or convenience. Then you would use that list to guide you throughout the day – making it easier for you to check off each item one by one. Now apply that logic to a routine activity like taking medicine. If you have to take multiple medicines each day at a specific time – why not make it easier on yourself and use a medication management device?

Why is Medication Management Important?

Managing your medications is important for a successful recovery or continued management of a chronic illness or disease. Think about the facts: for seniors, who typically take more medications than those under the age of 65, it is even more essential to take the right medication, at the right time, and not mix them with anything that could cause an adverse reaction. Adults (65 years or older) are twice as likely to need emergency care for adverse drug reactions (with over 177,000 emergency visits each year) and nearly seven times more likely to be hospitalized after an emergency visit. If you take multiple prescriptions on a regular schedule, then using a medication management device such as automatic pill dispensers, alarm style reminders, and timer medicine caps can be helpful.

Automatic Pill Dispensers

Pill dispensers are portable devices that allow you to organize your medication by day/time. These devices provide safety and reassurance by dispensing the correct pills on a set day/time via an alarm/reminder mechanism. Most also lock when not in use, preventing the patient from taking the wrong pills, as well as preventing children from accessing the device. Average Cost: $70/pill dispenser

Alarm-Style Reminders

Alarm-style pill reminders typically have four alarm settings for morning, lunch, dinner, and bedtime to remind the user to take their pills. In addition to your typical alarms, some of these devices have recorded reminders such as, "Good morning. It's 9 AM and time to take your morning pills." These devices allow you to set daily alarms for desired dosage times, thereby making it easier to manage medications. Average Cost: $35/reminder device

Timer Medicine Caps

Timer medicine caps are digital timers with a count-up feature, which works like a stopwatch, automatically keeping track of how much time has passed since the medication was last taken. This will directly help with medication management since a user's first question is often, "When did I last take this medicine?" The cap also prevents a user from overtaking a medication. Average Cost: $7/per cap and bottle

The list above includes the main types of medication management devices, but there are others related to specific illnesses or needs as prescribed by your doctor. Other options, in addition to these devices, are mobile apps for medication management. If you are unsure about what device or app will be the best for you, do your own research and consider consulting a physician.

Medical Insurance

FIFTY-TWO

What is Medicare Part A and B?

Do you have, or are you considering signing up for Medicare? If so, it's important to make sure you understand the four different parts of Medicare to help prevent confusion and delay in getting the care you need. We just gave you a high-level overview of the four different parts. Now we're going to dive deeper into Medicare Part A and Part B, touching on who is eligible and what each does and does not cover.

Who is Eligible for Medicare Part A and B?

Medicare Part A (Hospital Insurance) and Medicare Part B (Medical Insurance) are available to those eligible, which include:

- Age 65+
- Disabled
- End-Stage Renal Disease (ESRD)

What is Medicare Part A?
Medicare Part A is for hospital insurance. This means that it

will help pay for many items that fall under hospital and facility costs. Items typically covered under Part A include:

- Hospital care
- Skilled nursing facility care
- Nursing home care
- Hospice
- Home health services

According to Medicare.gov, you usually don't pay a monthly premium for Medicare Part A coverage if you or your spouse paid Medicare taxes while working. This is sometimes called "premium-free Part A." If you buy Part A, you'll pay up to $413 each month in 2017.

What is Medicare Part B?

As noted above, Medicare Part B is for medical insurance. This means that it will help pay for medical costs outside of the hospital. Items typically covered under Part B include medically necessary services and preventative services such as:

- Doctor visits
- Clinical research
- Diagnostic testing
- Outpatient procedures
- Ambulance services
- Durable medical equipment
- Flu shots (or other vaccines)
- Mental health (outpatient, inpatient or partial hospitalization)

According to Medicare.gov, the standard Part B premium amount is $134 (or higher depending on your income).

However, most people who get Social Security benefits will pay less than this amount ($109 on average).

What is Not Covered by Medicare Part A or Part B?
Some items that you can anticipate not being covered by Medicare include:

- Long-term care
- Most dental care
- Eye examinations related to prescribing glasses
- Dentures
- Cosmetic surgery
- Acupuncture
- Hearing aids and exams for fitting them
- Routine foot care

In some cases, you may find Medicare will cover one of the items listed above, but you will most likely pay copayments, coinsurance, or a deductible. So always check with your physician, provider, and Medicare insurer before getting any procedures done. Keep in mind that the cost of Part A or Part B can vary if you do not sign up when eligible.

As you approach the age of 65, you should follow the steps outlined at https://www.medicare.gov/sign-up-change-plans/get-parts-a-and-b/when-how-to-sign-up-for-part-a-and-part-b.html to ensure you are enrolled on time and get the right coverage for your needs. Don't miss out on any healthcare coverage or savings. Share this with your friends and loved ones, so everyone is properly covered and understands Medicare Part A and Part B.

FIFTY-THREE

What is Medicare Part C?

Sometimes navigating Medicare feels like a math problem to solve; you must sign up for Parts A and B first, then you can get Part C to replace Parts A and B... confusing, right? Well, it doesn't have to be. Once you understand what Medicare is, and you've received an overview of parts A and B, it's time to dive deeper into Medicare Part C.

What is Medicare Part C?

Medicare Part C is often referred to as the Medicare Advantage Plan (or the MA Plan). Essentially, it is another Medicare health plan choice for a Medicare-eligible participant (aged 65+ or under special circumstances). Before explaining how it works and what it covers, you need to understand that you must have already enrolled in Part A (Hospital Insurance) and Part B (Medical Insurance) first – so keep that in mind as you contemplate the Part C option and if it is right for you.

Will the Medicare Advantage Plan (Part C) Replace Parts A and B?

If you join a Medicare Advantage Plan, the plan will provide all of your Part A (Hospital Insurance) and Part B (Medical Insurance) coverage. Additionally, Medicare Advantage Plans may offer extra coverage, such as vision, hearing, dental, and/or health and wellness programs. Most include Medicare prescription drug coverage (Part D), which we'll cover more in another blog.

What Companies Offer Medicare Advantage Plans?

Medicare Part C is offered through private health insurance companies. Medicare pays a fixed amount each month to these companies. The rules that are set for all parts of Medicare apply to the companies that provide Medicare Advantage Plans. Not sure where to find a company? The U.S. News and World Report published the best companies (by state) for 2017, available here.

What is Covered under Part C?

According to AARP, the following services are covered under Medicare Part C:

- All the benefits of Part A, except hospice care
- All the benefits of Part B
- Hospital stays
- Skilled nursing
- Home health care
- Doctor's visits
- Outpatient care
- Screenings and shots
- Lab tests

- Prescription drug coverage is included in many Medicare Advantage plans, but not all.
- Eyecare
- Hearing care
- Wellness services
- Nurse helpline

There may also be bundled extras depending on the plan.

This is a lot of information to take in. However, you shouldn't feel overwhelmed. There are plenty of resources out there to help you navigate the Medicare process.

FIFTY-FOUR

What is Medicare Part D?

Did you know that in 2016, roughly 41 million (of the 55 million people on Medicare) were enrolled in Medicare Part D (source)[3]? If 41 million people have it – you may be wondering what Part D is, and whether or not you should get it. So far, we've explained at a high-level what Medicare is and given a brief overview of its four parts which include Parts A and B (referred to as Original Medicare), and Medicare Part C (Medicare Advantage Plans). Here is more information about Medicare Part D – Medicare's Prescription Drug Benefit.

What is Medicare Part D?

Medicare Part D is the prescription drug benefit option for those already enrolled in Medicare Part A and/or B. It is a voluntary outpatient prescription drug benefit for those on Medicare. The plans are operated by private insurance companies that follow the rules of Medicare. If you want to get Part D coverage, you have to select this option and enroll in a private Medicare prescription drug plan (PDP) or a Medicare Advantage Plan with drug coverage (MAPD).

How Much Does Part D Cost?

According to the Center for Medicare and Medicaid Services (CMS), the 2017 Part D base beneficiary premium range is from $10-$100 per month. The costs for the drugs themselves will vary by the plan purchased and the cost of the prescription under that plan.

Can I Get Drug Coverage if I Opt Out of Part D?

Yes, if you are enrolled in a Medicare Advantage Plan (Part C), then you are able to receive prescription drug coverage. Through Part C coverage, you will have access to both medical services and prescription drugs. This is a good option for people who choose to receive all their Medicare benefits in one policy, usually through a health maintenance organization (HMO) or a preferred provider organization (PPO).

Under Part B, you are eligible for a limited set of drugs. Medicare Part B covers injectable and infusible drugs administered often by a physician and not at home.

How Do You Join a Medicare Drug Plan?

Visit the Medicare Plan Finder on Medicare's website – Medicare.gov. There you can review the plans available and make the best decision possible. Once you choose a Medicare drug plan (part C or Part D), you can join by:

- Enrolling on the Medicare Plan Finder or on the plan's website at https://www.medicare.gov/find-a-plan/questions/home.aspx.
- Completing a paper enrollment form.
- Call 1-800-MEDICARE (1-800-633-4227)

FIFTY-FIVE

What is Medigap?

Medicare (Parts A & B) provides coverage for hospital and medical insurance, but it does not cover everything. How can you fill in the missing coverage? A Medicare supplement plan, known as Medicap, can help you cover the costs you are responsible for directly. We've provided some background information below to help you understand if you should consider signing up for Medigap.

How Medigap Works

As we shared above, Medicare (Parts A & B) do not cover all medical expenses. As a result, some people are interested in supplementing their Medicare with additional insurance to provide coverage for:

- Medicare deductibles
- Coinsurance payments (copays)
- Hospital costs after the Medicare-covered days have been reached
- Skilled nursing facility costs after Medicare-covered days have been reached

Before you can purchase Medigap from a private insurance company, you must have already enrolled in Medicare Parts A & B. After you select a Medigap plan (also commonly referred to as Medicare Supplement Insurance or Med Supp), you will pay a monthly premium to cover items like the ones we listed above. Your payment to the insurer will then pay for most out-of-pocket expenses. This may cover the 20% coinsurance or copay required by Medicare. There are ten standard Medigap policies to choose from, named after various letters of the alphabet. Medigap A is the most basic "core" policy, offering 100% coverage for Medicare Part A coinsurance and hospital costs. Medigap policies only cover one person, so if both you and your spouse want Medigap coverage, you'll have to buy separate policies.

What Medigap Is Not

It is important to know that Medigap is not a Medicare Advantage Plan (which is Medicare Part C, and it replaces Parts A & B). In fact, you cannot enroll in Medigap if you have a Medicare Advantage Plan.

If you have a Medigap policy, you will have to drop it to move into a Medicare Advantage Plan. As we described in a previous section, "What is Medicare Part C," a Medicare Advantage Plan will provide all of your Part A (Hospital Insurance) and Part B (Medical Insurance) coverage. Plus, it may offer extra coverage, such as vision, hearing, dental, and/or health and wellness programs.

How to Search for a Medigap Policy

To search for a Medigap policy in your area, follow the instructions below:

1. Visit the Medigap search engine at https://www.medicare.gov/find-a-plan/questions/medigap-home.aspx
2. Enter your zip code and health status
3. Once filled in, click continue
4. You will then have a screen filled with the policies in your area, estimated cost, and a profile of the benefits offered.
5. Next, you can click on the companies *offering Medigap policy* which you can then contact directly

Do your research on what plans provide the right coverage at the right price for you. Explore the coverage in your area and discuss with your physician, as well as providers.

FIFTY-SIX

What is the CMS Chronic Care Management Program?

The Centers for Medicare and Medicaid Services (CMS) created a way for Medicare patients to receive more frequent personalized care outside of the doctor's office.

The program is called Chronic Care Management (CCM). Under this program, Medicare can reimburse primary care physicians $43.12 per patient/per month for spending at least 20 minutes in non-face-to-face consultations. Find out what CCM is, who is eligible, and what this change means for primary care physicians.

What is Chronic Care Management?

CCM is the continuous care of a patient that has chronic conditions (i.e., dementia, diabetes, etc.) from dedicated health care professionals through constant communication, increased access to care outside the doctor's office, system-based approaches for patient assessments, coordination of care and the general ability to access expert care. The CCM program, which is provided by CMS, offers financial incentives for primary care practices to provide the much-needed support for those with chronic conditions.

Who is Eligible to Receive CCM?

Medicare patients are eligible if he/she has multiple chronic conditions (two or more) that are expected to last at least 12-months or until death. These requirements open this program up to approximately 33 million Medicare beneficiaries since two-thirds of all Medicare beneficiaries have two or more chronic conditions, such as:

- Alzheimer's Disease
- Asthma
- Cancer
- Chronic Obstructive Pulmonary Disease
- Diabetes
- Heart Failure
- Hypertension
- And many others

Who is Eligible to Provide CCM?

Those eligible to provide the CCM through Medicare are physicians and non-physician practitioners including:

- Certified nurse-midwives
- Clinical nurse specialists
- Nurse Practitioners
- Physician Assistants

What Is the Impact for Primary Care Physicians?

The program is still in its infancy but based on a survey

(source)[4] of 45,000 American primary care physicians who treat Medicare patients, 67.33% of respondents are unaware or not familiar with the program (Smartlink Mobile). More than 50% of respondents are planning to launch a CCM program in their practice within a year. The program does offer great financial incentive for care, but some challenges include:

- Enrolling eligible patients
- Lack of staff/expertise to meet the 20 minutes monthly minimum for enrolled patients
- Maintaining an auditable record of time and tasks performed
- Meeting the electronic requirements

Physicians need to continue to enroll CCM patients into the program. Moving forward, it is clear that educating both the eligible patient population and the health care professionals on what is available will lead to increased enrollment and use of this program.

If you are an eligible Medicare patient that has two or more chronic conditions, speak with your physician today to explore the option of Chronic Care Management.

FIFTY-SEVEN

What is Long-Term Care Insurance?

We buy insurance because we cannot predict the future. Insurance protects us from unexpected things like car accidents, weather damage to the house, or for when goods are lost or stolen. The same thinking has been applied to healthcare and the long-term care we may need as we age. Long-term care insurance (LTC) was created in the early 1990s to help provide coverage for care typically not covered by health insurance, Medicare, or Medicaid. The information below will provide you with additional information on what LTC is, who is eligible, how to get it, and what it can cost.

What is LTC (Long-term Care Insurance)?

As you age, you may find that you need help with dressing, bathing, or other activities of daily living (ADLs) due to a decrease in mobility or a physical or mental disability. Such needs are often not covered by traditional health insurance (including Medicare). This is where long-term care can help. Long-term care insurance provides benefits for those with functional or cognitive impairment. By purchasing a long-term care policy, you will pay to receive benefits (or reimbursement) for the long-term care costs associated with:

- Bathing
- Dressing
- Transferring (into and out of bed/chair)
- Toileting
- Eating
- Incontinence

These long-term care benefits can be provided at various caring locations including:

- At-home
- Assisted Living Communities
- Continuing Care Retirement Communities (CCRCs)
- Skilled Nursing Facilities
- Other care facilities

Who is Eligible for LTC?

In general, if you are in good health and over the age of 18, you can most likely find long-term care insurance. It is easier to look at what is excluded from coverage which includes in most cases:

- Mental and nervous disorders or diseases
- Alcoholism and drug addiction
- Illnesses caused by an act of war
- Treatment already paid for by the government
- Attempted suicide or self-inflicted injury

How Can I Get Long-Term Care Insurance?

If you are interested in LTC, you should contact your current insurance provider to see if it is offered. Outside of the private insurers, you can look into your Area Agency on Aging to see if any state or local options are available.

What Does Long-Term Care Insurance Typically Cost?

Each plan's cost will vary based on the coverage required. The cost is calculated based on the following:

- Your age at the time of purchase
- The maximum dollar amount the policy will pay per day
- The maximum number of days (years) that a policy will pay
- Additional benefits you choose with the policy

For example, a policy for a typical couple in Maryland in good health, aged 50+, can have an initial cost of $3,100 annually. Based on a recent review by the AARP, it is important to note that the premiums can shoot up without warning. The typical benefit amount ranges from $50 to $250 per day (source)[5]. To put the option of long-term care into perspective, only 8 million people currently have long-term-care coverage in the U.S., and only 131,000 policies were purchased in 2015 (down 24% from 2013) (source)[6]. Many people choose not to buy long-term care insurance. Instead, they save for their future long-term care needs on their own and pay for any necessary care out of pocket.

As you can see, the option of getting long-term care is available for most people. However, it is not widely used and can be confusing to obtain and get reimbursed. Make sure you do your homework, contact an insurance provider, and get all of your questions answered before deciding if LTC is right for you and/or your aging loved one.

FIFTY-EIGHT

Do You Need Long-Term Care Insurance?

"We had LTC insurance and had been paying the premiums for four years. The premiums have gone up 35% in that time, so we canceled!! As we are in our mid-fifties, we decided to cancel it and put that money in our retirement fund instead. Full-time nursing care runs $17,000/month in my area. No joke. My mom is in that facility, on Medicaid. No other way to do it. Less and less insurance companies are offering LTC policies because more and more people are using their LTC insurance, and it just isn't profitable to the insurance companies anymore. If we decide to get it later, we will pick a policy that has an equity portion."

Without question, we will all face additional costs to care for ourselves or for aging loved ones. How we pay for those long-term care costs (nursing home care, at-home care, etc.) is what should be planned out ahead of time. One option is Long-Term Care (LTC) Insurance.

If you get LTC insurance, you will be reimbursed for common day-to-day activities, but you must first demonstrate you have lost the ability to engage in at least two activities of daily living (ADLs) which are: eating, bathing, dressing, toileting, walking, and continence. After making sure you fully understand what Long-Term Care insurance is, it's important to understand what experts say about it, what the costs and benefits are, and what alternatives are available in order to decide if it is right for you.

What the Financial Experts Say

Many financial experts suggest that Long-Term care insurance is not a smart investment if you pay more than 5% of your monthly income on it. Since the launch of LTC insurance for consumer consumption, many experts have found that many policyholders have been unable to continue paying their premiums due to increasing cost. Premiums can rise at any point in time and are not fixed (like Life Insurance). Also, many of those who purchased LTC insurance and then lived at a nursing facility were unable to collect any reimbursement because they could still perform their ADLs. Lastly, many of the LTC benefits that were paid were often less than the actual cost of care (source)[7].

What You Pay for Long-Term Care

The annual cost for LTC insurance can range from $3,000 – $6,000 depending on a variety of factors, such as sex, age, health status, maximum daily benefit, length of benefit, and waiting period. Those premiums can go up in yearly increases of 3% to 5% (source)[8]. Keep in mind that you may start paying for LTC in your 50's, but may not need it until your late 60's or 70's.

What You Get from Long-Term Care

A strong LTC policy may cover at least $300/day. This type of policy may have inflation protection, which often only lasts for three years. The volatility in healthcare costs may limit the value of $300/day in 10-20 years from now. The coverage offered through LTC can provide, in many cases, more than Medicaid and can include anywhere from 24-hour care in your home (or at a facility) to just a few hours a week in at-home care.

What Are the Alternatives to Long-Term Care

To determine what coverage you will need, first determine how much you will have in your retirement savings and income. Based on that, you can calculate the cost of care in your area using the Cost of Care calculator from Genworth. Using the anticipated cost in comparison to your future income and assets will help you identify what (if any) difference exists. Based on your findings, discuss what options will work best for you with your financial advisor.

How to Know if LTC is Right for You

In the end, you need to make the right choice based on your personal circumstances. To get started, follow these steps:

- Do your own research and don't fall for any sales pitches
- Compare policies and all of the benefits offered from each one
- Read and understand the fine print in each policy

- Ask all of your questions upfront and write down the answers
- Understand and research each company
- Search for any consumer reports on the policy offered
- Do not buy what you cannot afford
- Apply early and plan for the future
- Think about your spouse in each policy
- Discuss and review this topic every single year

What we do know is the future is unpredictable, but we can plan to put ourselves in the best financial position possible. Discuss all options available and choose what is right for you and your loved ones.

FIFTY-NINE

The Best Long-Term Care Insurance Companies

As you age, you may find that you need help with dressing, bathing, or other activities of daily living (ADLs) due to a decrease in mobility or a physical or mental disability. Such needs are often not covered by traditional health insurance (including Medicare). This is where long-term care can help. Long-term care insurance provides benefits for those with functional or cognitive impairment. If you aren't sure, check out our blog Do You Need Long-Term Care Insurance?

If you want to better educate yourself on Long-Term Care options prior to speaking with one of the following groups, we highly recommend the book by Joseph Matthews: Long-Term Care: How to Plan & Pay for It. It delves into this complicated topic in an easy-to-understand manner. It is currently in its 12th edition and is a good value to help you understand your options. If you have decided that long-term care insurance is right for you, then use the list of the top 10 companies below, provided by ConsumersAdvocate.org, to get started.

The Top Ten Long-Term Care Insurance Companies

Golden Care
GoldenCare Long-Term Care Specialists work one-on-one to educate you on all of your coverage options and to help guide you in your LTC planning. All of their products are hand-selected from top-rated carriers in the long-term care insurance industry. GoldenCare specialists have more than 40 years' experience in long-term care insurance.

LTC Resource Centres
LTC Resource Centers is an independent Managing General Agency that has been providing solutions to chronic health care needs (dependency) for over four decades. Their product portfolio includes; long term care insurance, short-term care, linked or combo products, Medicare supplements, life insurance, critical illness, and annuities.

LTC Financial Solutions
LTC Financial Solutions, LLC is composed of long-term care specialists with over 65 years of experience. LTC Financial Solutions, LLC specialists make searching for long-term care insurance easier by assisting clients find long-term care solutions that are tailored to their needs. It educates clients about the benefits of long-term care insurance and helps them find a plan that matches their budget.

CLTC Insurance Services
CLTC Insurance Services provides long-term care solutions all over the nation by shopping all insurance companies for the best options and discounts available for your unique situation. The company also offers a Free Planning Guide, a "no obligation" consultation, and multiple quotes presented by one

expert agent dedicated to helping you make the right choice to protect, you, your family and assets.

ACSIA Partners

ACSIA Partners LLC is a company that offers a variety of long-term care and related insurance products across the country. At ACSIA Partners, your quotes are delivered by one single specialist, who helps you choose the best features and discounts, without over-buying coverage. Avoid mistakes when planning your long-term care policy with one-on-one guidance from ACSIA Partners.

Mutual of Omaha

Mutual of Omaha offers a large amount of policies and plans that are designed to meet individual needs and budgets. These come with different features that ensure your long-term care plan is able to handle future needs. You have the option to choose how to receive policy benefits.

New York Life

New York Life is a leading financial service provider backed by its strong capital position. It is one of the largest mutual life insurance companies in the country today and is rated A++ by AM Best. With its strong financial ratings, the company is positioned to be a reliable company for its long-term care customers now and in the future.

MassMutual

MassMutual is one of the biggest and leading insurance providers in the country today. The company enjoys high financial scores from some of the most credible financial rating sites that include AM Best, Moody's, and S&P. With good financial standing, the company is poised to provide long-term care insurance services well into the future.

Northwestern Mutual

Northwestern Mutual is a rock-solid provider of long-term care insurance with sound financial backing. The company offers a comprehensive list of plans and benefits that are up to par with the best plans being offered today. Northwestern Mutual offers automatic inflation-protection at 3, 4, and 5%. This means that a similar plan without inflation-protection, which provides $100 daily benefit, could be enhanced to $200 daily benefit with inflation-protection.

Genworth Financial

Genworth Financial offers a range of products and services, including long-term care insurance and mortgage insurance. In 2016, the company suspended sales of annuities and life insurance, putting the existing books of business into runoff. In 2012, Genworth's U.S. companies paid over $3.2 billion in benefits to life insurance, long-term care insurance, and annuity policyholders and beneficiaries. The company provides individual long-term care insurance, group long-term care insurance for employers offering benefits to employees, and caregiver support services.

TransAmerica Long-Term Care

TransAmerica offers a variety of financial services and is considered as one of the top insurance services in the country today. The company aims to make long-term insurance more available by providing a myriad of solutions that includes tax-qualified and inflation-protected plans to make LTC more affordable and effective.

If you choose to get LTC insurance, you will be reimbursed for common day-to-day activities, but you must first demon-strate you have lost the ability to engage in at least two activi-ties of daily living (ADLs) which are: eating, bathing, dressing, toileting, walking, and continence.

If you've decided to purchase long-term care insurance, make sure to take your time and research each of the companies listed above.

Legal Concerns

SIXTY

What to Do When Financial and Legal Issues Arise

"Knowledge is power." This old adage is true in many circumstances, but potentially none more important than when responding to an emergency involving the health of a loved one. Having access to information – regarding medical history, available benefits, assets, bills, important contacts, etc.– can make or break a family's ability to support each other in a crisis. Taking the time while the sun is shining to gather important information, and to ensure accessibility of that information by appropriate individuals, can greatly increase efforts to respond to a future storm.

What Information Should Be Gathered?

In order to ensure that trusted family members and/or friends have the information they need to step-in and help effectively when it would be helpful or necessary, the following information should be readily available:

- **Original estate planning documents:** The legal authority family members and friends have to assist in an emergency situation is granted by the formal estate planning documents (e.g., Trusts, Wills, Powers of Attorney, and Advance Medical Directives). As a result, it is critical to ensure that such documents are readily accessible.

- **Skeletal List of Assets:** In order to ensure that bills can be paid and finances can be managed, it is important to document the landscape of financial assets/accounts, including:
- Location of checking/savings/brokerage/retirement accounts, etc.
- Information regarding health/life/long-term care insurance policies
- **Roster of Important Contacts:** It will be important for the individuals stepping-in to help to be able to connect with various resources, including:
- Professional advisors (e.g., CPA, financial advisors, estate planning attorney, etc.)
- Medical professionals
- Other family members and friends
- **Letter of Guidance to Decision-Makers & Family Members:** Any specific wishes in connection with the following issues should be clearly documented:
- Medical care
- Management of financial affairs
- Funeral arrangements
- Cremation/burial arrangements
- Desired disposition of items of tangible personal property

Where Should this Information be Stored?

In order to preserve the security of the information and to ensure that it is easily accessible when needed, care should be taken when selecting the location(s) in which it is stored. Consideration should be given to the following:

- Original estate planning documents (e.g., Trusts, Wills, Powers of Attorney and Advance Medical Directives) should be stored in a secure location, such as a safety deposit box or fireproof safe.
- Copies of the estate planning documents, as well as the other information listed above, can be:
- Delivered to the individuals who will be stepping in to help in an emergency (e.g., individuals listed in the estate planning documents)
- Stored in a central location accessible to the individuals who will be stepping in to help in an emergency
- Kept safe by a third party instructed to release the information to the proper individuals in an emergency
- Stored electronically (e.g., cloud-based storage solution)

Taking time to proactively and deliberately gather and store critical information, and ensuring accessibility of that content, can enable family members and friends to feel empowered and in control in what otherwise could feel like a helpless situation. Do not delay – do it today.

SIXTY-ONE

What Legal Authority Do I Need to Access My Parent's Financial, Legal, or Health Records?

If you have not already, you should have a discussion with an attorney and your parent(s) about setting up a general power of attorney, durable power of attorney, joint account, trust, or advance directive. One (or all) of these documents will give you the legal authority to make decisions and obtain the legal, financial, and medical documents necessary to take care of your parent(s).

Why Do I Need Written-Legal Authority to Access my Parent's Information?

The primary reason you will need written legal authority to access your parents' documents is the Health Information Portability and Accountability Act (HIPAA). HIPAA keeps a person's health information and records private. Unless your parent gives you written authorization to receive that information, it is illegal for doctors to share any details with you about your parent's health.

What Legal Authority Should I Establish?

There are several types of authorities needed to properly manage and obtain your parent(s) legal, financial, and health-care affairs. Below is a brief summary of some of the available authorities:

- **Health-Care Proxy:** a legal document that names a health care agent. The health care agent will not only have decision-making powers but also have full access to confidential medical records.
- **Advance Healthcare Directive:** written instructions regarding an individual's medical care preferences. The forms vary from state to state, but in general, advance directives can include a Living Will, Health Care Power of Attorney or Health Care Proxy, and Do Not Resuscitate or Do Not Intubate Order (DNR or DNI).
- **Durable Power of Attorney:** is a document that grants a person or persons ("Attorney-in-fact") the legal powers to perform on behalf of the elder ("Grantor") certain acts and functions specifically outlined in the document. This power is effective immediately and continues, even if the grantor becomes disabled or incompetent. The powers usually granted include real estate, banking and financial transactions, personal and family maintenance, government benefits, estate trust, and beneficiary transactions.

For a complete list, contact a legal adviser.

Why Are These Authorities Important?

At some point, your parent may not be able to manage their own legal matters and will rely on you to act in their best interest. Planning ahead allows your parent and your family to have the legal authority to make critical decisions. If these authorities are not established prior to your parent becoming incapacitated, then you or another family member must ask a court to appoint a conservator or guardian, which may be a more complicated and difficult process.

To establish any of the authorities listed above you, should contact a professional legal adviser immediately.

SIXTY-TWO

What is an Elder Law Attorney?

Are you sometimes confused when reading about Medicaid, wills and trusts, what it means to be a guardian, or legal power of attorney? There are both online and in-person resources available to help make these topics less complicated. One of those resources is an elder law attorney. This may be a new term for you, so we have outlined some background information on the role of an elder law attorney, what one can do for you, and how to find one in your area.

What is an Elder Law Attorney?

Elder law attorneys are lawyers that handle a variety of legal issues specifically related to older or disabled adults. Elder law attorneys can act as advocates for those they represent. These legal matters can include items such as:

1. Healthcare
2. Long-term planning
3. Guardianship
4. Medicare/Medicaid

These experts can handle important financial and estate planning matters. In addition, due to their unique role and experiences, they can help with common issues that impact the care of seniors, like assisted living and end-of-life planning.

What Can an Elder Law Attorney Do for Me?

An elder law attorney can help you in many ways. Some of the common areas in which caregivers may need legal assistance, advice or enlist the support of an attorney on behalf of their care recipient include:

- Representation of the guardian on legal and financial matters as needed
- Guidance and creation of durable power of attorney, trusts, or estate planning
- Planning for Medicare or Medicaid coverage
- Processing social security and disability claims
- Probate avoidance
- Elder abuse and fraud recovery
- Understanding health and mental health law
- General guidance and assistance with long-term care planning
- And much more

How to Find an Elder Law Attorney Near You

To search for an attorney near you that has specialized experience in elder care law – visit the National Elder Law Foundation and search for a Certified Elder Law Attorney (CELA) and follow the instructions below:

- Visit www.nelf.org/find-a-cela
- Select your state by clicking on it

- Search through the list provided by the location nearest you

The legal scenarios faced by older adults can become more complicated when social security, Medicare, and estate planning are involved. An elder law attorney may be the support you need. Do some more research on your own and contact an attorney if you feel it would be helpful to you.

SIXTY-THREE

How Can I Know If My Family Needs More Estate Planning?

By Dan Vaughan, Esq., Kathi Ayers, Esq.

One of the biggest mistakes people make in the area of estate planning is to incorrectly assume they do not need to put a plan in place. This leaves a large portion of the population in either an unprotected or under-protected position, and because a lack of planning does not produce negative consequences until an emergency arrives, they are often not aware of this planning gap. A critical step to making sure your family has all of the protection it needs is gaining an understanding of the main areas of risk, so you can confirm that protections are in place to eliminate or minimize the effects of those risks.

Do I Need More Estate Planning?

By answering the following questions, you will be able to determine your need to consult with an estate planning professional to create estate planning solutions to protect your family:

- Is a plan in place to ensure that trusted individuals are empowered to assist with financial, administrative and medical decisions in the event of an illness or accident?
- Have steps been taken to ensure that assets will pass to beneficiaries following death without being exposed to the time, expense, and hassle of court-supervised probate?
- Are there planning measures in place to ensure that the proper beneficiaries receive the proper assets upon death? If so, does that plan address issues such as the incapacity or death of a beneficiary prior to distribution, and distribution to a beneficiary who may not be ready to manage the assets he or she will be receiving (e.g., until a younger beneficiary attains a certain age)?
- If you total the value of all of the assets (including life insurance policies and retirement accounts), can you say with certainty that the current value is less than the Federal estate tax exemption ($5,450,000 in 2016) and that the value, when added to any estimated future growth (including potential inheritances), will not exceed that figure in the future? If not, have you put a plan in place to address potential Federal estate tax liability?
- If local/State estate taxes are relevant (i.e., if the applicable local/State law is one of 15 jurisdictions that imposes a separate local/State estate tax in certain circumstances), can you say with certainty that the value of all of the assets is less than any applicable local/State estate tax exemption (e.g., $675,000 in New Jersey in 2016)? If so, can you say with certainty that the value of the assets, when added to any estimated future growth (including potential inheritances), will not exceed that figure in

the future? If not, have you put a plan in place to address potential local/State estate tax liability?

- If children from different marriages are involved in the planning, is a plan in place to guarantee that each of the children from the respective marriages will receive the inheritance intended for him or her?
- If any of the intended beneficiaries have special needs and/or are eligible for Federal and/or State assistance, is a plan in place to ensure that the distribution of assets to such beneficiaries will not cause complications and/or result in ineligibility to receive benefits?
- If a small business is in the picture, is a plan in place to ensure the appropriate transition of ownership in the event of incapacity or death and to ensure that the beneficiaries receive proper value for the business interest upon the occurrence of either of those events?
- If sizable gifts to any beneficiaries are desired, has an estate planning professional been consulted to ensure that the gifting goals are accomplished while achieving the most tax-effective transfer of such property to such beneficiary(ies)?

While these questions do not uncover every possible planning need, they address the most common core issues provided for in a comprehensive estate plan.

If you've answered "no" to any of the questions above, you should consider consulting with an estate planning professional to ensure that proper planning is in place to meet all of your needs.

SIXTY-FOUR

Caregiving Resources Offered Through the Workplace

Being a caregiver is difficult enough but add a 40+ hour work-week and you will definitely be in need of some extra help. Did you know that some workplaces offer Caregiving resources to their employees? Below are some important workplace resources that your employer may be offering.

Workplace Caregiving Resources

The U.S Equal Employment Opportunity Commission (EEOC) outlines best practices for employers to ensure that there are no violations against workers who are also caregivers. These examples of resources illustrate the growing demand on caregivers at work, impacting both the employee and employer. In addition, the Family & Medical Leave Act (FMLA) does provide certain employees with up to 12-weeks of unpaid leave, which includes caring for a spouse or parent with a serious health condition.

To learn more about what your company can do for you as a Caregiver, start by having a discussion with your supervisor and asking about the following questions:

- **Does your office allow for flextime:** this could include the option of working 40 hours during the week but not during the standard 9 am – 5 pm (i.e., working long hours one day and less the next).
- **Does your office offer advanced annual or sick leave?** - this could help in preparing for any time off needed for caring for someone after surgery or other needs.
- **Does your office allow for telework?** - offices are becoming mobile now and working from home, or other remote locations is becoming easier and easier with new technology.
- **Does your office allow for a leave of absence (or leave without pay)?** - this could be helpful if you need a specific amount of time (6-9 months as an example) to care for a loved one or to assist your family during bereavement enabling you to keep your position available when you return.
- **Does your office have an employee assistance program (EAP)?** - depending on the size of your organization, there may be a dedicated office that helps employees during challenges faced at work or at home from a supportive role.
- **What state-specific laws exist to help caregivers at work?** - each state may have specific legislation protecting caregivers.

This important subject has both the Federal government and private sector employers working towards solutions. One such coalition is ReACT (Respect A Caregiver's Time), which is made up of 75+ employers from corporations, colleges, non-profits, and government entities. The mission of ReACT is to create a supportive business environment where the challenges faced by caregivers, juggling the demands of both work and caregiving for an adult with a chronic age-related disease, are understood and recognized by employers so that employees can better meet their personal and professional responsibilities.

If you're a Caregiver, it's important to learn about all of the resources available to you. These are just a few questions to discuss with your supervisor or Human Resources department directly. The suggestions above are to help you prepare for the conversation and know your rights as an employee and as a Caregiver. Be willing to compromise and find what will work best for you, your employer, and your family. Do your research and be open-minded when discussing this sensitive subject with your employer.

SIXTY-FIVE

What is Probate and How Can it be Avoided?

By Dan Vaughan, Esq., Kathi Ayers, Esq.

"I was executor of my grandmother's estate in 2002, and before that basically helped my mom take care of legal things when my dad died. Both times, having a properly executed will naming me (or my mother) as executor was all that was needed to handle financial affairs posthumously."

Estate Planning is the process of legally structuring the future disposition of current and projected assets (Forbes) and is an important part of End-of-Life planning. Unfortunately, when Estate Planning isn't put in place prior to a parent's passing, their adult children can find themselves unprepared and unexpectedly thrown into the Probate process, which can be time-consuming, expensive, and very stressful. Given that this process is optional, you should consider creating an estate plan while your parent is living so you can bypass the probate process.

What is Probate?

Probate is the legal process that local governments use to ensure that assets properly pass through a deceased person's estate. In other words, the court ensures that the decedent's debts are paid off and that any remaining assets are given to the correct beneficiaries. On the plus-side, probate does provide accountability and transparency to the estate administration process. However, that benefit comes with material costs such as court-related taxes and fees and professional accounting and legal expenses.

When is Probate Required?

There is a common misconception that probate is only required if a decedent died without a Last Will and Testament and that by creating a Will and ensuring that assets pass through the Will upon death, the probate process will be avoided. Unfortunately, the opposite is true. Sending the assets through a Will is what requires probate. Anytime assets pass through a decedent's Will (whether the decedent created the Will himself or herself, or the Will is supplied by state statutory law, because he or she did not create a Will) probate is required in order to permit the court to supervise the process and to protect the interests of the estate's creditors and beneficiaries.

What Are the Disadvantages of Probate?

The following are disadvantages of Probate:

- **Joint ownership with rights of survivorship** –

any asset owned jointly with rights of survivorship automatically passes to the surviving joint owner(s) following an owner's death.

- **Beneficiary designation** – any asset that has a valid beneficiary designation (e.g., life insurance or retirement accounts) is payable to the named beneficiary(ies).

- **Revocable trust** – any asset owned by (or payable by beneficiary designation to) a revocable trust is distributed pursuant to the terms of the trust.

How Can Probate be Avoided?

Because probate only applies to assets passing through a deceased person's sole name through his or her estate, it can be avoided by ensuring that every asset is controlled by one of the following distribution alternatives:

- **Joint ownership with rights of survivorship** – any asset owned jointly with rights of survivorship automatically passes to the surviving joint owner(s) following an owner's death.

- **Beneficiary designation** – any asset that has a valid beneficiary designation (e.g., life insurance or retirement accounts) is payable to the named beneficiary(ies).

- **Revocable trust** – any asset owned by (or payable by beneficiary designation to) a revocable trust is distributed pursuant to the terms of the trust.

Each of these tools has a different subset of pros and cons, so it is important to consult with an attorney to fully understand which works best to accomplish your goals.

Do I Still Need a Will?

Even if you intend to avoid probate by using joint ownership, beneficiary designations and/or a revocable trust, it is still important to have a Will to act as a safety net to catch any assets that may have been overlooked. In addition, a Will is also important for individuals with minor children, as the Will is where guardians for those children are appointed.

In order to streamline the time and expense associated with the distribution of assets following death, consult with a legal advisor to evaluate whether your estate plan should be constructed in a manner that avoids the probate process.

SIXTY-SIX

In the News: President Passes the RAISE Family Caregivers Act

President Trump recently signed the Recognize, Assist, Include, Support, and Engage (RAISE) Family Caregivers Act into law. The passage of this law is a very positive sign that despite many political disagreements, there is overwhelming bipartisan support of caregivers across this country. We've provided a brief summary about this law and its implications below.

What is the RAISE Act?

In summary, this law directs the Department of Health and Human Services (HHS) to develop and a National Family Caregiving Strategy that is publicly available and identifies recommended actions for recognizing and supporting family caregivers in a manner that reflects their diverse needs. In addition, the HHS shall convene a Family Caregiving Advisory Council to advise the department on how best to recognize and support family caregivers. The department will have 18 months to develop its initial strategy and then must provide annual updates.

What Can You Expect from the RAISE Act?

"Family caregivers are the backbone of our care system in America. We need to make it easier for them to coordinate care for their loved ones, get information, and resources, and take a break so they can rest and recharge," said Nancy A. LeaMond, AARP's chief advocacy and engagement officer. The outcome of the bill and the advisory council will identify and recommend actions that communities, providers, government, and others are taking and may take to recognize and support family caregivers, including with respect to:

- Promoting greater adoption of person and family-centered care in all health and Long-Term Services and Supports (LTSS) settings, with the person and the family caregiver (as appropriate) at the center of care teams
- Assessment and service planning (including care transitions and coordination) involving care recipients and family caregivers
- Information, education, training supports, referral, and care coordination
- Respite options
- Financial security and workplace issues

All caregivers and supporters should recognize this as a good sign. With that said, pay close attention to all legislation that impacts you as a caregiver. We should hopefully see the positive impact of the RAISE Act in the years to come.

Financial Concerns

SIXTY-SEVEN

What Financial Documents Do I Need to Keep for My Aging Parents?

As your parents get older, you will want to make sure you keep their critical financial documents organized. Obtaining and retaining these documents will give you the information you need to protect your parents' financial assets. However, how do you know which documents are important to hold onto?

What Financial Documents Should Be Kept?

The National Institute on Aging provides a great list of critical financial documents that should be kept. Consumer Reports expands in more detail on this financial paperwork:

Essential records:
Keep birth and death certificates, marriage licenses, divorce decrees, Social Security cards, and the two most recent tax returns. Credit and debit card names and numbers. Investment income (stocks, bonds, property) and stockbrokers' names and phone numbers. Any bank statements.

Defined-benefit plan documents:
Keep pension-plan documents from your current and former

employers. Also include the sources of income and assets (pension from your employer, IRAs, 401(k)s, interest, etc.)

Estate-planning documents:
Keep copies of wills, trusts, and powers of attorney. Last mortgage payment, as well as when the payments are due. Location of the original deed of trust for home and car title and registration. The most recent appraisal and property tax document (including any house/condo records).

Insurance Information:
Keep insurance information (life, health, long-term care, home, car) with policy numbers and agents' names and phone numbers. For permanent life insurance—policies that have a cash value or investment component. Include any Medicare and/or Medicaid documentation.

Discussing Finances with Your Parents

The information listed above should be stored in a location so that key people know where to find them (i.e., family, lawyer, etc.). To start, you should compile a list of everything above, where each item is located, and include as much detail as possible. Ask your parents the following questions to understand what types of financial documents they may have and note the location of any/all financial documents:

- Where do you store your financial documents?
- Do you have a safe deposit box? If yes, where is it and where is the key?
- Where is the most up-to-date will with an original signaturelocated?
- What are the names of your banks and account numbers (checking, savings, credit union)?

- Do you have an accountant or financial planner? If yes, what is his/her contact information?

Take the time to understand what documents are critical to retain and others that may be more clutter than beneficial. Review the list of key financial documents, gather the information, provide the relevant detail, and store the information in the best place that makes the most sense for you.

SIXTY-EIGHT

Three Ways Family Caregivers Can Become Financially Secure

Currently, more than 40 million Americans are providing unpaid long-term care services to family members and loved ones. Dubbed as everyday superheroes, these individuals dedicate a big portion of their time, health, and financial resources to provide the best care possible to their aging loved ones. In doing so, they put themselves and their individual futures at risk. One of the biggest risks of being a family caregiver is the danger of losing financial resources to support their own needs. So what can family caregivers do to take control of their finances? In order to find fiscal security, while mitigating the potentially devastating financial impact, caregivers should think about long term care, seek out deductions and discounts.

How Much Are Caregivers Spending?

At this point, it is considered common knowledge that long term care services can cause a severe blow to anyone's finances. In fact, AARP released a report stating that family caregivers dedicate approximately 20% ($6,954) of their annual income to cover out-of-pocket care services. Now that the increase in the cost of living has overtaken income growth by 13%, family caregivers find themselves in a tough position financially.

Consider Long Term Care

One of the many questions associated with long term care is this: is long term care insurance necessary or not? More importantly, will family caregivers benefit from securing a policy? To answer these questions, we need to get a good look at what caregivers go through in the process of providing care. Yes, they are often quoted describing the role as rewarding and fulfilling, but how has the responsibility impacted various aspects of their lives?

In a separate study, AARP shared the following data:

- One in five caregivers experiences financial problems and high levels of physical strain.
- Two in five caregiver experiences emotional stress, especially those who work a high number of hours.

With this in mind, the long-term care needs of these family caregivers may just be around the corner. As they shoulder a big portion of their care recipient's expenses, they might find that they do not have enough money to fund their own out-of-pocket care expenses.

Without proper coverage—one that was secured early while they were healthy—these caregivers might end up relying on their own adult children too, and thus starting a crippling cycle. Long term care insurance premiums may be daunting now, but with the sky-rocketing costs of care services, it may be better to be safe (and covered) than sorry.

Seek Out Deductions and Discounts

In a post by the Association for Long Term Care Planning on ALTCP.org entitled, Family Caregiver Duties: Effective Financial Planning, caregivers are advised to look into long term care tax deductions. Here are some tax tips, as well as benefits that maybe be available to Caregivers. To qualify, caregivers must be able to claim that their care recipients are their dependents and that they are either citizens of the US or residents of the US, Canada, or Mexico. Moreover, they must be able to prove that they are shouldering at least half of their parents' expenses. The detailed list of requirements is indicated on the IRS website.

Utilize All Available Resources

Some family caregivers have had to leave their jobs to meet the high demands of care. Although some situations may call for this action, family caregivers must think carefully and consider all options first. Leaving a job does not just cut off a steady source of income; it also means putting a stop to a sizable chunk of employer-sponsored retirement plans and contributions to Social Security. Make sure you seek out all of the Caregiving Resources that may be offered through your workplace.

In order to make sure that care recipients still get the services that they need, family caregivers should also look into services offered for free or at a discounted price in their local communities, as well as their local faith communities. Services offered may include meal delivery, transportation, respite, or day programs.

SIXTY-NINE

The Cost of At-Home Dementia Care

We are always trying to understand the true cost of being a caregiver and estimate that the aggregate of lost wages, pension, and Social Security benefits of those serving as caregivers to their parents is nearly $3 trillion.

Even more shocking is that the total health care costs related to dementia care are more than $287 billion annually in the U.S alone. So how does this apply to you? If you are a caregiver for a loved one with dementia, you should expect some unexpected costs. The most significant driver in dementia costs is the fact that the disease is treatable but not curable.

We'll describe the common costs you can anticipate for at-home dementia care below in more detail. Use this information to help you prepare financially or decide if there are other options besides home-care that meet your needs.

Common Costs for At-Home Dementia Care

To be financially prepared to care for a loved one with dementia, please make sure you are familiar with the answers to the following FAQ's:

What are the out-of-pocket costs for caregivers? You can expect to spend at least $10,000 each year on various costs supporting your loved one, such as prescription drugs, personal supplies, adult care services, safety-related expenses, and more.

What are the out-of-pocket costs for your loved one? According to a 2015 study in the Annals of Internal Medicine, the average cost for your aging loved one will be $61,500 in out-of-pocket expenses annually. This is compared to $34,068 for those without dementia.

What are the costs of a dementia (or memory) care facility? The costs can vary but generally range from $3,165 to $5,800 per month (source).

What do professional at-home care services costs? The costs can vary based on your location and needs, but the average cost starts at $21/hour.

What are the estimated prescription drug costs? The average prescription drug costs for dementia care are $3,000 per year, which is three times what someone with Medicare pays (source).

How much do safety and tracking devices cost? Tracking your loved one can be done with a mobile app, a wearable GPS tracking device, and/or a remote monitoring device.

What additional medical costs can you expect? Dementia care will typically cost more than more routine and time-limited care. You can expect increased costs associated with memory care training and additional caregiver support.

You need to be prepared for the costs associated with at-home dementia care as best you can. You can't anticipate when and if this will happen to you, but understanding the costs will help you make the best decisions when it comes to your loved one's care.

To help pay for these costs, form a plan with the input of other family members as well as professionals. Keep in mind that someone with dementia can live for many years. Do the math and see what works best for everyone.

SEVENTY

What is the True Cost of Caregiving?

If you are suddenly faced with the prospect of providing care for a loved one, you are likely unaware of the costs involved with caregiving. According to MetLife, the total estimated aggregate lost wages, pension, and Social Security benefits of those serving as caregivers to their parents is nearly $3 trillion. There are numerous costs you can expect and need to plan for. However, you also need to plan for the unexpected, hidden costs of being a caregiver.

What Are the Costs of Caregiving?

For those working and serving as a caregiver, the loss of wages can be as drastic as the following:

- For women:
- The total individual amount of lost wages due to leaving the labor force early and/or reduced hours of work because of caregiving responsibilities equals $142,693.
- The total impact of wages, retirement benefits, and social security equals $324,044.

- For men:
- The total individual amount of lost wages due to leaving the labor force early and/or reduced hours of work because of caregiving responsibilities equals $89,107.
- The total impact of wages, retirement benefits, and social security equals $283,716.
- See the full MetLife Study here. (source)[9]

Other than lost wages, the cost of caregiving can include various out-of-pocket expenses, such as:

- All of the out of pocket expenses below can cost a caregiver approximately $4,570 to $8,728 per year (according to an Evercare and National Alliance for Caregiving study):
- Household goods
- Food and meals
- Travel and transportation costs
- Medical care co-pays and pharmaceuticals
- If needed, home renovation expenses to accommodate mobility issues for your parent can cost on average $6,226. Read more about home renovation costs here.
- If required, hiring additional, professional home caregiver support can cost on average $21 per hour.

The largest financial impact on a caregiver can be the loss of wages as a result of having to take time off of work. This can also impact your employability down the road.

The cost of being a caregiver can be great. To prepare yourself for these costs, you should research what tax benefits are available for you as a caregiver, as well as additional support if you or your loved one is a veteran. Discuss these costs with your family and budget properly for the expected and unexpected costs of being a caregiver.

SEVENTY-ONE

Out-Of-Pocket-Costs for Family Caregivers

Earlier, we discussed the true cost of caregiving, in which we highlighted the reported loss of wages over a lifetime (upwards of $140,000 for women). We also presented that the possible out-of-pocket costs ranged from $4,570 to $8,728 per year. Until just recently, that was the extent of available research on the subject. However, a recent AARP research study dug even deeper into the extent of out-of-pocket costs and provided specific detail on what you can expect to spend on out-of-pocket caregiving related expenses (source)[10]. Below is our summary of the findings of that study.

The Out-of-Pocket Expense of Caregiving

During the study, AARP found that "family caregivers spend an average of $6,954 on out-of-pocket costs related to caregiving, nearly 20% of their annual income." This is a significant dollar amount, and it is consistent among caregivers. Caregiver out-of-pocket expenses typically include:

- Household goods
- Food and meals

- Travel and transportation costs
- Minor (or major) home modifications

These types of costs are about 41% of expenses. Another 25% of out of pocket expenses include medical care co-pays and pharmaceuticals.

The Impact of Out-of-Pocket Costs

Taken directly from the report, the following breaks down the variation of expenses by ethnic groups and other scenarios, in order by dollar value:

- Asia-Americans/Pacific Islanders spent $2,935
- African-American family caregivers spent $6,616
- White family caregivers spent $6,964
- Caregivers who shared the same home spent $8,616
- Hispanic/Latino family caregivers spent an average of $9,022
- Caregivers for those with dementia spent $10,700
- Long-distance family caregivers (defined as those who lived more than an hour away) spent $11,923

These are costs coming directly out of your bank account, every year. Keep in mind that if your annual expenses are $10,700, in five-years that will equal $53,500. That is a significant cost that can severely impact your day-to-day life, as well as what you had saved for your own future. So, what can you do to prepare?

- Plan out all anticipated expenses for your aging loved one
- Put together a budget and timeline of these expenses
- Get help from a financial advisor

- Utilize caregiver financial assistance options that are available to you
- Keep track of your expenses and evaluate regularly

You need to be prepared and know what out-of-pocket expenses you can expect. Don't wait until it is too late. Start discussing options with your family, aging loved one, and financial advisor today.

SEVENTY-TWO

Are There Tax Benefits Available for Caregivers?

Most people are well-aware of the daunting costs involved with providing care to older parents or family members. However, many people involved in the process of providing this care don't realize that there are numerous ways to recover many of these expenses in the form of tax benefits. For example, did you know that when you file your taxes you may claim deductions and credits for a range of out-of-pocket expenditures such as:

- Dental treatments
- Cost of transportation to get to a medical appointment
- Health insurance premiums
- Long-term care services

And there is more. If you are a family caregiver, you can find other creative ways to claim exemptions and other deductions. Find out more below.

Exemptions for Dependents

Many people don't realize that dependency exemptions can also apply for older Americans under the care of family members. You may claim a dependency exemption for U.S. citizens if:

- You provide more than 50% of a person's living costs
- The dependent is a family member or lives in your primary residence
- the dependent does not jointly file a tax return with another person
- The dependent does not have income that exceeds the current exemption amount (this amount can change annually). This scenario is quite common and can provide a tax exemption of $4000.

Tax Deductions for Medical Expenses

If you are currently paying for medical costs for a parent or relative, you can also include those with your other expenses for your personal tax deduction. In most cases, this applies whether your parent or relative qualifies as a dependent or not. These expenses can also include certain long-term care costs of an infirm individual. These savings can end up being quite significant if your costs are high.

Tax Credits for Dependents

If your parent or relative is unable to care for his or herself, you may also be eligible for a tax credit for a portion of costs that limit you or your spouse's ability to work. This credit is only available if your family member lives with you.

These are just a few of the current tax breaks available to

individuals involved with eldercare. This information is provided as general information and should not be treated as professional or advice. In addition, many states have additional tax deductions or tax credits to provide financial relief to caregivers. Please consult a qualified tax and or legal advisor.

SEVENTY-THREE

In the News: Credit for Caring Act Looks to Save Your Tax Dollars

In May 2017, the Credit for Caring Act was introduced in the U.S. House and Senate. The purpose of the proposed bill is to amend the Internal Revenue Code of 1986 to provide a nonrefundable credit for working family caregivers.

The bill (if passed) would increase the available tax credit for family caregivers up to $3,000 in a taxable year. This tax credit would provide eligible family caregivers caring for loved ones of all ages with some financial relief and help them pay for services such as in-home care, adult daycare, respite care, and other support services. To help provide some context and background information, we've highlighted some key elements of the bill below.

What will the Credit for Caring Act Do?

The act would help save family caregivers money by offering a federal tax credit of up to $3,000. This bill would amend the IRS Code to allow an eligible caregiver a new tax credit for 30% of the cost of long-term care expenses that exceed $2,000, up to $3,000 in a taxable year. The bill defines "eligible caregiver" as an individual who has earned income for the taxable year in excess of $7,500 and pays or incurs expenses for providing care to a spouse or other dependent relative with long-term care needs.

Who Introduced the Bill?

Senators Joni Ernst (R-IA), Michael Bennet (D-CO), Shelley Moore Capito (R-WV), and Elizabeth Warren (D-MA), and Representatives Tom Reed (R-NY) and Linda Sánchez (D-CA) introduced the bill in the House and Senate respectively. A similar bill was proposed during the last congressional year but did not make it to a vote.

How Can I Track the Bill?

The title of the bill is the Credit for Caring Act. In the Senate, the bill number is S. 1151 and H.R. 2505 in the House. You can check for status updates at Congress.gov (https://www.congress.gov/bill/115th-congress/house-bill/2505).

Who Would be Eligible for the Tax Credit?

According to an AARP summary of the bill, family caregivers must meet the following criteria to receive the tax credit:

- Be a spouse, adult child, parent or another relation named under the "dependent" definition
- Help a loved one, of any age, who meets certain functional or cognitive limitations or other requirements, as certified by a licensed health care practitioner
- Have more than $7,500 in earned income for the taxable year
- Able to document qualified expenses

Family caregivers spend an average of $6,954 on out-of-pocket costs related to caregiving each year. These out-of-pocket costs are exactly why caregivers need as many tax breaks as possible. Pay close attention to H.R. 2505 and S.1151 – the Credit for Caring Act 2017 as it may benefit you directly.

SEVENTY-FOUR

What is the Special Compensation for Assistance with Activities of Daily Living (SCAADL)?

Our veterans and service members deserve the best care and support possible, especially during the transition from active service to discharge. To provide that, the Department of Defense (DoD) established the Special Compensation for Assistance with Activities of Daily Living (SCAADL). For those eligible, SCAADL can provide relief of the financial burden that caregivers face when caring for veterans needing non-medical care, support, and general daily assistance for up to 90 days after discharge.

What is SCAADL?

As described directly by DoD – the 2010 National Defense Authorization Act authorized the Special Compensation for Assistance with Activities of Daily Living.

This special monthly compensation is for eligible catastrophically injured or ill service members who require assistance with daily living activities or who are at high risk for personal safety and therefore cannot live independently in the community without caregiver support.

SCAADL provides financial assistance for the non-medical care, support, and assistance by a primary caregiver for the service member. This is a taxable special monthly compensation. It is paid directly to the service member to help offset the primary caregiver's loss of income.

The monthly compensation will range based on the required amount of time the daily service is needed (10 to 40 hours a week) and is calculated by using the U.S. Department of Labor's Bureau of Labor Statistics wage rate for home health aides. Some examples include:

- Bethesda, MD, (Tier 1) minimal support needed = $644/month
- Austin, TX, (Tier 2) medium support needed = $1,780/month
- Detroit, MI (Tier 3) maximum support needed = $2,180/month

For a monthly estimate in your area visit: http://militarypay. defense.gov/Calculators/SCAADL-Calculator/.

Who is Eligible for SCAADL?

Those eligible for SCAADL must, at a minimum:

- Have a catastrophic injury or illness incurred in the line of duty;
- Have been certified by a licensed physician to be in need of assistance from another person in order to perform the personal functions of everyday living; or
- Would, in the absence of this provision, require some form of residential institutional care.

This specific caregiver compensation was designed to support service members and caregivers before, during, and 90 days after the transition/discharge date.

How Do You Apply for SCAADL?

This offering of financial support is not automatic for veterans who are eligible and need it. You must apply directly with the DoD for this compensation. If you think you or the veteran you care for may be eligible, have your physician fill out the DD Form 2948 and send it to your Wounded Warrior Regiment for review and processing.

Looking for more veteran benefits? Continue reading on for our list of the top benefits and resources available.

SEVENTY-FIVE

Caregiving Benefits for Veterans: The Top Benefits and Resources Available

Did you know that there are more than 12.4 million veterans 65 years and older living in this US? The Federal government provides a range of benefits for these veterans and their caregivers. Below is a list of those benefits and resources available.

What Benefits are Available for Older Veterans?

Older veterans have numerous options available through the Veterans Administration and may be eligible for the following:

- **Geriatrics and Extended Care Services (GEC):** is committed to optimizing the health and well-being of veterans with multiple chronic conditions, life-limiting illness, frailty or disability associated with chronic disease, aging or injury.
- **Home and Community-Based Services:** These services help chronically ill or disabled veterans of any age remain in their homes. You can receive more than one service at the same time.
- **Residential Settings and Nursing Homes:**

These services include community residential care, assisted living, and community nursing homes.

- **Aid & Attendance and Housebound Benefit for Veterans:** is an increased monthly pension amount paid if you meet the eligibility requirements. Learn more about it here.

- **Program of Comprehensive Assistance for Family Caregivers of Veterans:** This benefit provides certain medical, travel, training, and financial benefits to caregivers of certain veterans and service members who were seriously injured during service on or after September 11, 2001. Learn more from about it here.

To learn more, you should contact a VA regional office and discuss these benefits with an employee to determine if you are eligible, how to fill out the forms, and what steps you need to take.

What Resources are Available for Caregivers of Veterans?

Caregivers of veterans will need support from within and outside their community. There are a number of resources available for the caregivers to find support, including:

- **Department of Veterans Affairs' Caregiver Support Line:** The support line can discuss assistance available from the VA, help access services, answer questions about eligible services, or connect caregivers with the Caregiver Support Coordinator at the closest VA Medical Center. To contact, call: 1-855-260-3274

- **Department of Veterans Affairs' Caregiver Support:** This website provides resources for caregivers and Veterans, including resources available to caregivers, and videos and stories of caregivers of Veterans. The website also has a zip code lookup feature, allowing caregivers and Veterans to find the name and contact information of the closest Caregiver Support Coordinator.

- **Veterans Health Library:** This website provides information on common health issues faced by veterans, including information related to caring for a Veteran with a specific illness, injury, or condition.
- **Department of Veterans Affairs' Guide to Long Term Services and Supports:** This website provides an overview of VA long-term services and supports.
- **Respite Care:** This is designed to relieve the family caregiver from the constant burden of caring for a chronically ill or disabled veteran at home. Services can include in-home care, a short stay in an institutional setting, or adult day health care.
- **Dental Care Resources for Veterans:** Emergency Dentists has put together a guide that provides information on everything you need to know about dental care for active duty and retired veterans.

The best place to start is researching the information above and contacting the VA Caregiver support line to learn more. You can call 1-855-260-3274 to learn more about caregiver and veteran support available. We need to care for our older veterans, and the best way to begin is by being prepared and knowledgeable of all resources and benefits available.

Research and Prevention

SEVENTY-SIX

In the News: Dementia Rates Decrease in the U.S.

We want to share with you some encouraging and hopeful news. A recent study has found that between 2000 and 2012, the rate of dementia in the United States decreased from 11.6% to 8.8%. To put it into perspective, if the rates remained constant, then there would be one million+ more people with dementia than there are today (source). This significant decline brings hope and shines a light on the positive work being done by scientists, researchers, physicians, and patients.

Study Summary

In this study, published by JAMA Internal Medicine, the question that was asked was, "Has the prevalence of dementia among older adults in the United States changed between 2000 and 2012?" The study used data from two specific years (2000 and 2012) and looked at more than 10,000 Americans who were at least 65 years old. In 2000 – 11.6% of them had some form of dementia. In 2012 – 8.8% had dementia. That is a significant decrease!

Although it is not definitive, the result of the study identified the following as the primary influences:

1. The primary influence cited is education. The impact of education, both in years of schooling, as well as the easy access to new and challenging information, is linked to the decrease in dementia.
2. Those aged 85+ had an increased body weight than in 2000. This can provide more nutrients and energy to help the brain maintain cognitive function.
3. The risk of cardiovascular disease (a known cause of dementia) has decreased. The disease has been at the forefront of public awareness campaigns aiding in this decline.

The next step for searchers is to try and definitively understand why there has been a decrease.

How Can You Actively Work to Prevent Dementia?

As suggested by recent research, we know that the function of the brain (no matter its age or status) can be improved by taking a holistic approach and making specific adjustments in your lifestyle. The holistic approach, which has been broken down into five key cornerstones of daily living, (Move, Discover, Relax, Nourish, and Connect) and has been well documented and researched by the AARP and supported through several additional studies.

The continued focus on caring for our aging population has shown its value with a decrease in the number of those with dementia. We must continue this fight by actively pursuing new research, working in our own ways to prevent dementia, and raising awareness among your loved ones.

SEVENTY-SEVEN

In the News: Bill Gates and the Dementia Discovery Fund

The Dementia Discovery Fund (DDF) is a global effort bringing together funding from the private sector, charity, and industry from all over the world.

The Dementia Discovery Fund (DDF)

The DDF is a venture capital fund which invests in projects and companies to discover and develop novel, effective disease-modifying therapeutics for dementia. Seven leading pharmaceutical companies (GSK, Biogen, Lilly, Takeda, Pfizer, Johnson & Johnson, and Astex, a subsidiary of Otsuka), the UK's Department of Health, and charity Alzheimer's Research UK have invested in the DDF to date. Managed by SV Life Sciences Managers LLP, the DDF follows a mandate to validate novel hypotheses and expand the breadth of targets and mechanisms in development for dementia over the 15-year life of the fund.

Recently, Bill Gates invested $50 million in the DDF to accelerate progress towards disease-modifying therapies for Alzheimer's disease. This personal investment will help the

venture capital fund to bring together industry and government in order to seek treatments for severe memory loss.
Gates recently said, "[Dementia] is a huge problem, a growing
problem, and the scale of the tragedy – even for the people
who stay alive – is very high," he said. He went on to say, "I
believe we are at a turning point in Alzheimer's research and
development, in which the Dementia Discovery Fund is
playing an important role by exploring new approaches to
treat the disease. I'm excited to join the fight and can't wait to
see what happens next."

Dementia puts a significant demand on the caregiver's
emotional and financial wellbeing. This personal investment is
a significant sign that many other philanthropists will follow.
There is hope! With the help of the DDF and its network of
public/private partnerships, the outlook on dementia research
and discovery is quite positive.

SEVENTY-EIGHT

In the News: Preventing Alzheimer's May Become a Reality

Earlier we shared hopeful news that from 2000 to 2012 there was a decline in the rate of Dementia. We are excited to share some more encouraging news, provided by a recent 60-Minutes investigation called the Alzheimer's Laboratory. Researchers have found an extended family in Colombia with a genetic mutation that causes Alzheimer's. This discovery may help scientists prevent the disease someday, which could be a monumental shift in the future of Alzheimer's worldwide.

Clinical Trial Summary

60 Minutes reported that years ago, a young doctor and nurse in Colombia unraveled the mystery of many patients who were diagnosed with Alzheimer's disease in their mid-40s. The significant finding was that they were all a part of one large, extended family, connected generations back. As a result, a collaboration between public and private funding created a clinical trial study that scientists are hoping may help prevent the disease in others someday.

Why Is this Family Unique?

Many in this large family have a rare genetic mutation that causes early onset Alzheimer's. A genetic test revealed which relatives have the mutation, and they have been taking part in a study that began three years ago.

What is the Clinical Trial?

Genentech, the Banner Alzheimer's Institute, and the National Institutes of Health are collaborating on the first-ever prevention trial to be conducted on cognitively healthy individuals who have a genetic history of Alzheimer's Disease. The funding of the trial includes $15 million in research funding from NIH, $15 million from other philanthropists, and the remaining needs provided by a research and development (R&D) budget from Genentech. The Autosomal Dominant Alzheimer's Disease (ADAD) trial is currently focused on Colombia.

The trial focuses on prevention by using an immunotherapy drug to remove amyloid plaque, which is a known cause of Alzheimer's. From there, scientists place genetic biomarkers and have participants perform routine cognitive measurements to evaluate the participants before they show any symptoms of cognitive decline. As a result, the scientific community can monitor specific genes for changes and can mark those for continued study.

What is the Goal?

A simple genetic test could reveal which members of the family had the gene mutation that would guarantee they would get early onset Alzheimer's. "The question is," said Sean Bohen, Genetech's Senior Vice President of Early Development, "if we intervene before cognitive function deteriorates, can we prevent the disease?"

As recommended by 60-Minutes, for more information, visit the Alzheimer's Prevention Registry, a registry anyone 18 years or older can sign up for. Do your part and continue to follow and support Alzheimer's research.

SEVENTY-NINE

How to Improve Your Brain Health

"My father is 103, is physically healthy, and does not have dementia or Alzheimer's. When he was in Rehab after falling, the occupational therapist asked him questions every day to stimulate his brain to form new neural pathways to help his memory."

As you age, you will see natural changes in your skin, hair, and even mobility. How you age, however, depends on your genes, environment, and lifestyle (which includes personal choices). Another natural change that is taking place as you grow older, although not so visible to the eye, is how your brain functions. In order to stay healthy, active, and independent, it is imperative that you keep your brain healthy and/or improve brain health by integrating five key cornerstones into your daily life.

What is Brain Health?

According to the Administration for Community Living, brain health is the ability to remember, learn, plan, concentrate, and maintain a clear and active mind. Your brain health can be affected by your genetic makeup, diseases (such as Alzheimer's), brain injuries, smoking, poor diet, lack of sleep, and lack of physical activity.

How to Improve Your Brain Health

As suggested by recent research, we know that the function of the brain (no matter its age or status) can be improved by taking a holistic approach and making specific adjustments in your lifestyle. The holistic approach, which has been broken down into five key cornerstones of daily living, has been well documented and researched by the AARP and supported through several additional studies. The good news is, you can take immediate action, using the approach outlined below:

Move

Physical activity is associated with a lower risk of cognitive decline, according to the Alzheimer's Association. By exercising, you are immediately increasing the blood flow – and the flow of oxygen – to your brain and throughout your body. This is just what your brain needs, as the brain receives about 15-20% of the body's blood supply and survives on the oxygen supplied via the blood flow. Through exercise, you are able to also reduce stress, improve your memory, improve your sleep, and reduce blood pressure.

Discover

Challenging your brain by learning a new skill, a new subject, or hobby will have short and long-term benefits. It is important to continue to expose yourself to new challenges rather than routine actions (such as doing the same game repeatedly). "Cognitive and social engagement have been shown to be *protective* against cognitive decline, whereas hearing loss, depression, and social isolation are *associated* with cognitive decline," says Dr. Kathryn Papp, a neuropsychologist and instructor in neurology at Harvard Medical School.

Relax

You need to find ways to reduce stress, get enough sleep, and allow time for meditation. Your brain does not shut off when it is asleep and needs the time to refresh for the next day. By meditating, you can reduce your stress, calm your mind, and increase your ability to discover new things and challenge your brain. It has been reported that chronic stress can directly damage the brain, which reinforces the need to find time to relax your brain, find time to exercise, and find more *me*-time.

Nourish

The right diet will help give you energy to exercise and can also help you sleep. Your brain needs healthy fats from fish, berries, and other veggies that provide the right nutrients (such as Omega 3). Research suggests that the right foods and wrong foods can directly affect our physical and mental health. The Society for Neuroscience has found that "Our brains are sculpted by what we eat. If it's too much fat, too much sugar, or just too much [of anything', there may be permanent consequences for our brain function. Keeping our brains in shape is one more reason to clean up our diets."

Connect

Being social and participating in activities with others is associated with reduced risk for depression and can possibly delay the onset of dementia. John Cacioppo, a neuroscientist at the University of Chicago, researched loneliness in his book, *Loneliness: Human Nature and the Need for Social Connection*, outlining that social connections with others are essential for a long and healthy life. These social connections directly connect with our brain health and overall well-being.

The five cornerstones for brain health outlined above are your guide to get started. You may need to jump on all five, or just add only one or two into your regular routine. Discuss this topic with your loved ones and with your physician. Wherever you are in your journey, you can start today by incorporating all of these into your lifestyle to help keep your brain healthy and sharp.

End of Life Care

EIGHTY

Discussing End-of-Life Care

Emotionally, it may be a difficult conversation, but it is necessary, and you will thank yourself later if you know your loved one's wishes. To some, this may sound like a morbid thing to discuss; however, these types of discussions are extremely important. To help you get started, follow our four-step plan to discuss end-of-life care with your aging parents.

How to Discuss End of Life Topics

When you discuss end-of-life topics, you will need to broaden your scope away from resuscitation and other specific medical issues. In addition to those topics, you need to discuss fears, concerns, what everyone's goals and needs are, and the physical needs that will have to be considered. By doing so, you will open up lines of communication, help to mitigate or avoid conflict, and minimize fear and pain.

Plan Ahead and Avoid Surprises

Planning to have these conversations during the holidays gives you time to prepare and provides you with a comfortable setting. With that said, don't keep this a secret. The last thing you want is to spring this on your aging parents or anyone else in your family. Be open with everyone that you want to have this conversation. Explain what your expectations are and start by making sure that everyone is open to it. Maybe they are already thinking about having a conversation like this. Just like you, they may not know where to start. For the family meeting, you can outline the following agenda:

- Initiate the conversation by opening up with ground rules (be honest, be open, and listen)
- Clarify the goals of the conversation
- Have the discussion
- Develop an action plan

Include Everyone That Needs to Be There

Who should be a part of this conversation besides you and your parents? Your siblings? Grandchildren? Close friends? Make sure to include everyone that needs to be included. Be mindful of having too many people present at once. Remember, there can be multiple conversations and sharing of information afterward.

Put the Action Items and Plan in Writing

It's one thing to talk about what you need to do or want to do, and it is another to write it down. By putting your discussion in writing, you can assign tasks, create due dates to get legal and financial documents written and signed, and have a reference point. This should not be the last conversation you have on the topic of end-of-life care.

Be Open and Know Others Will Help

You need to be open to the idea that others can help. This means that you will share responsibility for your aging parents' end-of-life care. That can be a hard thing to share even with siblings, but remember that they want to help as well. Be open with your loved ones about your concerns.

End-of-life care and planning for it includes everything from financial planning to spiritual conversations. You cannot get to everything in an-hour but starting the conversation will open up future dialogue around a difficult topic. Break the silence on a hard topic and help everyone by initiating the conversation.

EIGHTY-ONE

What is Hospice Care?

"I am so overwhelmed. I flew to the Caribbean two days ago with my mother, to basically give palliative care to my gran, 83, whose kidneys are shutting down (8%). This is horrifically emotionally draining and exhausting. She's not eating at all, her body is becoming toxic, and we all know this is the end. Recommendations not to put her in a hospital as it is palliative, and could literally be any minute...or a month."

Caring for a loved one that has a life expectancy of six months or less can be emotionally draining and logistically complicated for all involved. However, you can find help and relief through hospice. Hospice is a specialized type of care for those facing a life-limiting illness, as well as their families and caregivers. Review the information below to help you determine if and when your aging loved one may need hospice care.

What is Hospice Care?

Hospice caregivers help to control pain in order to provide peace, comfort, and dignity to the recipient of care as much as possible. Hospice programs also provide services to support the family as well. Hospice supports patients with a terminal illness and their families by providing services such as:

- Pain management and help with problems breathing or swallowing
- Routine visits by a nurse or hospice staff
- Medication and other medical supplies
- Overall coordination of a patient's needs and care with in-home and hospital support
- Emotional and spiritual support for the patient, family, and caregivers

Overall, hospice focuses on caring, not curing, and in most cases, care is provided in the patient's home.

What a Hospice Care Team Looks Like

You and your family members are the most important part of a team that may also include:

- Doctors
- Nurses or nurse practitioners
- Counselors
- Social workers
- Pharmacists
- Physical and occupational therapists
- Speech-language pathologists
- Hospice aides

- Homemakers
- Volunteers

Consult with your physician and your insurance provider about the need for hospice care, or hospice options. The services available are there to help and guide you through a difficult time.

Discussing end-of-life care options can be difficult for many. To help you get started, follow our four-step plan to discuss end-of-life care with your aging loved ones, which can be found in the next section of this book.

Caring Village Resources

EIGHTY-TWO

Doctor's Visit Checklist

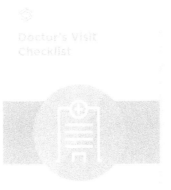

www.caringvillage.com/checklists/doctors-visit

EIGHTY-THREE

Caregiving 101 Checklist

Just-in Time
Caregiving Checklist

www.caringvillage.com/checklists/caregiving-101

EIGHTY-FOUR

Four Ways the Caring Village Family Caregiver Guide Checklist Can Help You

---

When you become a caregiver, there is no fanfare or fireworks. Instead, caregivers like you have been thrust into an unknown reality overnight that forces you to ask a lot of questions and compile a lot of information very quickly. However, the most significant and challenging questions are – Where do I start? What do I do first? This is where the free Caring Village Family Caregiver Guide Checklist can help you and your family.

Caring Village's Family Caregiver Guide Checklist

Our Family Caregiver Guide Checklist will help you understand what important Financial Medical, Legal, and Estate planning documents should be created, obtained, and stored for you or a loved one.

Once completed, our checklist will give you tremendous peace of mind by assuring you that you have all that you need are and that you have honored your loved one's wishes.

The Family Caregiver Guide Checklist helps you:

Determine what contact information and key documentation you need to collect and categorize.

In a section of this book, experts from Vaughan, Fincher & Sotelo outlined the information you will need access to in case of an emergency. You will first want to begin with capturing all of the important points-of-contact. Getting together all of the information in one consolidated place before an emergency occurs can save time, money, and potentially lives.

Get your financial information organized.

Trying to get all of your loved one's financial information together can be very confusing and difficult. To get started, you need to know what questions to ask when discussing finances with your aging loved one. The types of questions you can ask about the financial documents you will need include:

- Where do you store your financial documents?
- Do you have a safe deposit box? If yes, where is it and where is the key?
- Where is the most up-to-date will with an original signature located?
- What are the names of your banks and account numbers (checking, savings, credit union)?
- Do you have an accountant or financial planner? If yes, what is his/her contact information?

Get your legal and medical information consolidated and organized.

Do you know your parents' blood type? What allergies they have? What medicines are they taking? These are some of the questions you will have to answer when using this checklist.

Organizing your aging loved one's legal and medical information will put you in a good position to answer difficult questions from a doctor or insurance company.

Ask questions and find items you have never thought to inquire about.

When was the last time you talked to your parents about Irrevocable Life Insurance Trusts? You most likely haven't. That is just one of the multiple checklist items you will be charged to confirm in the Legal and Estate Planning portion of the Guide.

As a caregiver, you will be challenged to know a lot of information and learn it quickly. Knowing where to begin is the hard part, but we make it easy!

EIGHTY-FIVE

Financial, Legal and Estate Planning Checklist

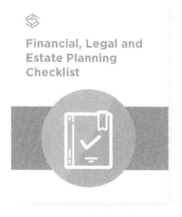

www.caringvillage.com/checklists/financial-medical-legal-estate/

EIGHTY-SIX

Home Preparedness and Maintenance
Checklist

**Home Preparedness
and Maintenance
Checklist**

www.caringvillage.com/checklists/home-safety

EIGHTY-SEVEN

Three Ways the Caring Village Home Preparedness Checklist Can Help You

As a caregiver, you will, or already have been, discussing whether your aging loved one will age in place or move in with you. The topic itself is difficult, and turning it into action can be overwhelming, complicated, and stressful. Where do you even start? This is where the Caring Village Home Preparedness Checklist can help make it easier.

Caring Village's Home Preparedness Checklist

The Caring Village Home Preparedness Checklist can help you prepare for this phase of your life by:

Showing you how to update all bedrooms, bathrooms, and kitchens to ensure they are safe for aging loved ones.

In a previous section of this book, we discussed how to prepare your house for elderly loved ones to move in by focusing on safety, mobility, and creating a smooth transition. To do all of this, you need to consider how these common rooms are safe for your loved one. Have you considered installing grab bars in the bathroom? Adding lights throughout the house? Installing a wheelchair ramp? Our checklist helps to lay out all that you need to consider.

Teaching you how to renovate bedrooms, bathrooms, and kitchens so that they accommodate those with limited mobility and/or are ADA compliant.

If your aging loved one currently has or is expected to have limited mobility, then you will have to accommodate their needs. There is a lot to consider when renovating any of your rooms for mobility restrictions. Have you considered the height of your cabinets? How heavy are your drawers and appliances? Should your loved one have bed rails? If you don't know how to answer these questions that is OK. Our checklist is meant to guide and help you through this process. It will ask the questions you did not consider.

Providing you with both indoor and outdoor General Home Maintenance Reminders

After you make the necessary changes to your or your loved one's home, there is still much to be done. You also need to routinely make changes and conduct seasonal maintenance to ensure your house is ready for the summer and winter.

In addition, don't forget to consider:

- The time it will take to purchase additional items (i.e., bed rails)
- Additional tools and supplies you may need to install or maintain certain items
- Contractors or technicians you may need to hire

Use our checklist to make getting a home ready for an aging loved one an easy and efficient process.

EIGHTY-EIGHT

TheSeven Best Books About Caregiving

Are you looking for a book about caregiving? If so, there are plenty of great ones out there. To help you narrow your focus, we've highlighted the six best books about caregiving below. These books have consistently ranked in the top five on a variety of caregiving websites and blogs within the past three years. Check out the books and descriptions below and let us know which one is your favorite.

The 7 Best Books About Caregiving

We start our list with a monthly highlight of **128 Days and Counting: A 28-Year Old Caregiver's Memoir** by Honore Nolting summarized by this customer review on Amazon.com: *"A wonderful book for anyone trying to better understand the multi-layer journey dealing with cancer and its aftermath. The author's humor keeps you entertained throughout while not diminishing the intensity of the situation. With cancer being something that touches far too many lives, this book does an amazing job helping individuals grasp what you could expect at each stage and offers insight to everyone involved (be it patient, caregiver, friend, family member). Take-home points for me being*

communication and support are key to survival, and the journey is unfor-
tunately not over when you hear "cancer free." Well done and good
luck, Honor and Tom!

"128 Days and Counting: A 28-Year Old Caregiver's Memoir" by Honore Nolting

128 Days is a vivid and detailed account of a young couple
during a cancer diagnosis and their relationship during the
most difficult time of their lives. Honore and her husband,
Tom, who went through chemo, an operation, and a difficult
adjustment period, come alive in these pages as a loving and
upbeat couple who are as familiar as your best friends. They
are strong and scared, normal and quirky, determined, and
silly. Excerpts from the blog written during Tom's cancer
answer many questions about what it's like to get cancer, and
be a caregiver, as young adults. Honore's raw and emotional
account about every aspect of the experience, and their relationship brings the reader fully into the magnitude of the
diagnosis but what lingers is the joy, resilience, and efferves-
cence of love.

"A Bittersweet Season: Caring for Our Aging Parents — and Ourselves" by Jane Gross

When Jane Gross found herself suddenly thrust into a caretaker role for her eighty-five-year-old mother, she was forced
to face challenges that she had never imagined. As she and her
younger brother struggled to move her mother into an assisted
living facility, deal with seemingly never-ending costs, and
adapt to the demands on her time and psyche, she learned
valuable and important lessons. Here, the longtime New York
Times expert on the subject of elderly care and the founder of
the New Old Age blog shares her frustrating, heartbreaking,

enlightening, and ultimately redemptive journey, providing us along the way with valuable information that she wishes she had known earlier. Learn why finding a general practitioner with a specialty in geriatrics should be your first move when relocating a parent; how to deal with Medicaid and Medicare; how to understand and provide for your own needs as a caretaker; and much more. Wise, smart, and ever-helpful, A Bittersweet Season is an essential guide to caring for aging parents.

"Can't We Talk About Something More Pleasant?" by Roz Chast, The New Yorker

In her first memoir, New Yorker cartoonist Roz Chast brings her signature wit to the topic of aging parents. Spanning the last several years of their lives and told through four-color cartoons, family photos, and documents, and a narrative as rife with laughs as it is with tears, Chast's memoir is both comfort and comic relief for anyone experiencing the life-altering loss of elderly parents. While the particulars are Chast-ian in their idiosyncrasies–an anxious father who had relied heavily on his wife for stability as he slipped into dementia and a former assistant principal mother whose overbearing personality had sidelined Roz for decades–the themes are universal: adult children accepting a parental role; aging and unstable parents leaving a family home for an institution; dealing with uncomfortable physical intimacies, and hiring strangers to provide the most personal kind of care.

"Caring for Your Parents: The Complete Family Guide (AARP)" by Hugh Delehanty

Drawing on AARP's deep wellspring of expertise in the topic, AARP's Caring for Your Parents offers both sensitive counsel and a practical road map through the complex emotional terrain many of us face as our parents age. This eye-opening book guides readers through a new, creative approach to caregiving that turns familial duty into a journey of emotional development and resolution.

Based on a 32-page National Magazine Award-nominated special feature, Caring for Your Parents documents the innovative ways that real people cope with this age-old issue. Throughout the book, you will find useful, field-tested recommendations from AARP's staff of experts. Topics explored in depth run the gamut from locating quality health care and dealing with the bureaucracy of Medicare to avoiding consumer scams, organizing caregiving from afar, and planning the disposition of an estate. There are tips on designing your parents' house to make it more elder-friendly, navigating the hidden dangers of assisted living, and dealing with the invisible sibling issue. A resource guide in each chapter lists helplines, websites, and consumer action groups.

"The Caregiver's Survival Handbook (Revised): Caring for Your Aging Parents Without Losing Yourself" by Alexis Abramson, PhD

Being a caregiver can be rewarding but demanding work-and more than 40 million adult children find themselves experiencing the double duty of caring for their elders as they try to carry on a life of their own. The mission of this book is to help caregivers figure out how to look after aging loved ones, provide for other family members, and attend to their own career-without losing themselves in the process. In this supportive, reassuring, and practical guide, Doctor Alexis addresses the most pressing concerns, including such issues as how to: Get all family members to pitch in; Let go of feelings of guilt; Avoid conflict with an aging loved one; Foster independence in the elderly; Balance the demands on one's own time and resources.

"AARP Meditations for Caregivers: Practical, Emotional and Spiritual Support for You and Your Family" by Barry J. Jacobs and Julia L. Mayer

Family caregiving has its challenges: emotional overload, time constraints, anxiety, burnout, missed work, adult sibling conflicts, and marital issues. AARP Meditations for Caregivers blends emotional and spiritual motivation to minimize the strains while helping caregivers view their work as a mission from the heart. Chapters are organized by theme, including topics such as accepting your feelings, knowing your limits, seeking support, and managing stress. Each reading offers a poignant meditation, an anecdote drawn from the author's personal or clinical experience, and hands-on or psychological advice to foster coping skills and a sense of fulfillment. The meditations in this indispensable book will provide you with solutions to typical caregiving challenges, offer relief and renewal through mindfulness, and inspire you to find meaning and value in the work you do.

"Don't Stop the Music: Finding the Joy in Caregiving" by Nancy Weckwerth

Based upon over twenty-five years of caregiving for Nancy Weckwerth's friend and partner, John D. Swan, the book describes how to find the joy in caregiving. Don't Stop the Music is a narrative of John's acceptance of his disability and Nancy's transformation to a caregiver. Nancy shares their journey through every triumph and challenge with honesty and openness. Her insights disclose the light, the lessons, and the laments that guided them across uncharted territory from surviving to thriving. Author Nancy Weckwerth has created a "survive and thrive" manual for Caregivers. The wisdom within is meaningful for any caregiving situation.

Pick up any or all of these books today!

.

Appendix & References

EIGHTY-NINE

Appendix

---

101 Mobility:
https://www.caringvillage.com/101mobility

ACSIA Partners LLC:
https://www.caringvillage.com/acsia

Administration for Community Living:
http://www.acl.gov

ADT – Home Alert System:
https://www.caringvillage.com/ADT

Alzheimer's Association Care Team Calendar:
https://www.alz.org/care/alzheimers-dementia-care-calendar.asp

Alzheimer's Association Care Training:
http://www.alz.org/care/alzheimers-dementia-care-training-certification.asp#elearning

American Heart Association:

http://cpr.heart.org/AHAECC/CPRAndECC/
FindACourse/UCM_473162_Find-A-Course.jsp

AngelSense Elderly GPS Tracker:
https://www.caringvillage.com/angelsense

Association for Long Term Care:
http://www.ALTCP.org

Bay Alarm Medical - Home Alert System:
https://www.caringvillage.com/BayAlarm

Bruno Stair Lifts:
https://www.caringvillage.com/bruno

Caregiver Online Group:
http://lists.caregiver.org/mailman/listinfo/caregiver-
online_lists.caregiver.org

Center for Medicare and Medicaid Services (CMS):
https://www.cms.gov

**Centers for Disease Control and Prevention (CDC)
Adult Vaccine Quiz:**
https://www2.cdc.gov/nip/adultimmsched

**Centers for Disease Control and Prevention (CDC)
Important Facts about Falls:**
https://www.cdc.gov/homeandrecreationalsafety/
falls/adultfalls.html

Centers for Medicare and Medicaid Services (CMS):
https://www.cms.gov/Outreach-and-Education/Medicare-
Learning-Network-MLN/MLNProducts/
Downloads/ChronicCareManagement.pdf

CLTC Insurance Services:
https://www.caringvillage.com/CLTC

Consumer Advocate:
http://www.consumersadvocate.org

Consumer Protection Safety Commission:
https://onsafety.cpsc.gov

Department of Defense (DoD):
https://www.defense.gov

Department of Health and Human Services:
http://www.hhs.gov

eCaregivers:
http://ecaregivers.com

EHLS, a Lifeway Mobility Company:
https://www.caringvillage.com/lifeway

Emergency Dentists:
https://www.emergencydentistsusa.com

Family & Medical Leave Act (FMLA):
https://www.dol.gov/general/topic/benefits-leave/fmla

Family Caregiver Alliance:
https://www.caregiver.org/women-and-caregiving-facts-and-figures

Family Caregiving Alliance Practical Skills Training for Family Caregivers:
https://www.caregiver.org/practical-skills-training-family-caregivers

Genworth Financial Long-Term Care Insurance:
https://www.caringvillage.com/genworth

GPS SmartSole:
https://www.caringvillage.com/smartsole

GoldenCare:
https://www.caringvillage.com/goldencare

GreatCall Medical Alert:
https://www.caringvillage.com/GreatCall

Health in Aging – Eldercare at Home:
https://www.healthinaging.org/aging-health-a-z

Home Instead Senior Care:
https://www.homeinstead.com/news/daughters-in-the-workplace

Improvement Center Stair Lifts:
https://www.caringvillage.com/improvementcenter

iTraq GPS Tracker:
https://www.caringvillage.com/itraq

LifeFone Medical Alerts:
https://www.caringvillage.com/LifeFone

LifeStation Medical Alerts:
https://www.caringvillage.com/LifeStation

Lotsa Helping Hands:
http://lotsahelpinghands.com

LTC Financial Solutions, LLC:

—

https://www.caringvillage.com/LTCFinancial

LTC Resource Centers:
https://www.caringvillage.com/LTCResource

MassMutual:
https://www.caringvillage.com/MassMutual

Medical Alert:
http://www.medicalalert.com

Medical Guardian – Home Alert System:
https://www.caringvillage.com/medicalguardian

Medicare Plan:
https://www.medicare.gov/find-a-plan/questions/home.aspx

Medicare.gov:
https://www.medicare.gov

MobileHelp:
https://www.caringvillage.com/MobileHelp

Mutual of Omaha:
https://www.caringvillage.com/mutualomaha

National Alliance for Caregiving:
http://www.apa.org/pi/about/publications/
caregivers/faq/statistics.aspx

National Association of Area Agencies (N4A):
http://www.n4a.org

**National Association of Professional Background
Screeners (NAPBS):**

http://www.napbs.com/resources/about-screening

National Association of Social Workers:
http://www.helpstartshere.org/helpstartshere/?
page_id=3677

National Council on Aging (NCOA):
https://www.ncoa.org/public-policy-action/elder-justice/
elder-abuse-facts

National Elder Law Foundation:
http://www.nelf.org

National Immunization Awareness Month (NIAM):
https://www.nphic.org

National Volunteer Caregiving Network:
https://nvcnetwork.org/wp/

New York Life:
https://www.caringvillage.com/NYLife

Northwestern Mutual:
https://www.caringvillage.com/NWMutual

**Nursing Home Law News: A Guide to Preventing
Elder Abuse:**
https://www.nursinghomelawcenter.org/news/nursing-home-
abuse/guide-preventing-elder-abuse

Philips Lifeline Medical Alert:
https://www.getphilipsmedalert.com

PocketFinder GPS Tracker:
https://www.caringvillage.com/pocketfinder

Respect A Caregiver's Time (ReACT):
http://respectcaregivers.org

Senior Corps:
http://www.nationalservice.gov/programs/senior-corps/
senior-companions

**Special Compensation for Assistance with Activities
of Daily Living (SCAADL):**
https://warriorcare.dodlive.mil/benefits/scaadl

Spy Tec GPS Tracker:
https://www.caringvillage.com/spytec

Stannah Stair Lifts:
https://www.caringvillage.com/stannah

The American Red Cross:
http://www.redcross.org/take-a-class/cpr

The Caregiver Training University:
http://www.caregivertraininguniversity.com

The Family Learning Center:
http://www.ipced.com/training-programs/family-learning-
center

The National Safety Council:
http://www.nsc.org/pages/home.aspx

Trackimo GPS Tracker:
https://www.caringvillage.com/trackimo

Trax GPS Tracker:
https://www.caringvillage.com/trax

TransAmerica Long-Term Care:
https://www.caringvillage.com/TransAmerica

U.S Equal Employment Opportunity Commission (EEOC):
https://www.eeoc.gov/policy/docs/caregiver-best-practices.html

Vaccines.com – Your Best Shot at Good Health:
https://www.vaccines.gov/diseases

Veterans Administration:
http://www.benefits.va.gov/persona/veteran-elderly.asp

VA Regional Office Lookup:
http://www.va.gov/directory/guide/
division_flsh.asp?dnum=3

Aid & Attendance and Housebound Benefit for Veterans:
http://benefits.va.gov/
pension/aid_attendance_housebound.asp

Dental Care Resources for Veterans:
https://www.emergencydentistsusa.com/dental-care-resources-for-veterans

Department of Veterans Affairs' Caregiver Support Line: (To contact, call: 1-855-260-3274):
http://www.caregiver.va.gov/support/support_services.asp

Department of Veterans Affairs' Guide to Long Term Services and Supports:
http://www.va.gov/GERIATRICS/Guide/
LongTermCare/index.asp

Geriatrics and Extended Care Services (GEC):
http://www.va.gov/geriatrics

Home and Community-Based Services:
http://www.va.gov/geriatrics/Guide/
LongTermCare/Home_and_Community_Based_Services.asp

Program of Comprehensive Assistance for Family Caregivers of Veterans:
http://www.caregiver.va.gov/support/support_benefits.asp

Residential Settings and Nursing Homes:
http://www.va.gov/geriatrics/Guide/
LongTermCare/Nursing_Home_and_Residential_Services.asp

Respite Care:
http://www.caregiver.va.gov/support/support_services.asp

Veterans Health Library:
http://www.veteranshealthlibrary.org

NINETY

References

1. **National Alliance for Caregiving (NAC) and the AARP Public Policy Institute.** *Caregiving in the U.S.* 2015 Retrieved from http://www.caregiving. org/wp-content/uploads/2015/05/ 2015_CaregivingintheUS_Final-Report-June-4_WEB.pdf
2. **Alzheimer's Disease International.** *World Alzheimer's Report: The Global Impact of Dementia*: 2015 Retrieved from https://www.alz.co.uk/research/ world-report-2015
3. **Henry J Kaiser Family Foundation.** *The Medicare Part D Prescription Drug Benefit*: 2017 Retrieved from https://www.kff.org/medicare/fact-sheet/the-medicare-prescription-drug-benefit-fact-sheet/
4. **Smartlink Health.** *Market Research Report: MACRA Success Strategies*: 2017 Retrieved from http://www. smartlinkhealth.com/resource-center/market-research-report-macra-success-strategies/
5. **National Association of Insurance Commissioners.** *Long Term Care Insurance Fact Sheet*:

2018 Retrieved from https://www.naic.org/
cipr_topics/topic_long_term_care.htm

6. **The Wall Street Journal.** *Long-Term Care Insurance:
Is It Worth It?* 2015 Retrieved from https://www.wsj.
com/articles/long-term-care-insurance-is-it-worth-it-
1430488733

7. **NOLO.** *Long-Terms Care Insurance: The Risks and
Benefits*: 2017 Retrieved from https://www.nolo.com/
legal-encyclopedia/long-term-care-insurance-risks-
benefits-30043.html

8. **CNBC.** *Weighing the Pros and Cons of Long-Term Care
Coverage*: 2015 Retrieved from https://www.cnbc.
com/2015/01/28/weighing-the-pros-cons-of-long-
term-care-coverage.html

9. **MetLife.** *Caregiving Costs to Working Caregivers: Double
Jeopardy for Baby Boomers Caring for Their Parents*: 2011
Retrieved from Retrieved from https://www.
caregiving.org/wp-content/uploads/2011/06/mmi-
caregiving-costs-working-caregivers.pdf

10. **Alzheimer's Association.** *Alzheimer's Disease Facts
and Figures Report*: 2016 Retrieved from https://www.
cbsnews.com/news/family-caregivers-spend-huge-
percent-of-income-on-care-costs-aarp-survey/

11. **Cancer Network.** *The Crisis of Cancer: Psychological
Impact of Family Caregivers.* 1997 Retrieved from
http://www.cancernetwork.com/review-article/
crisis-cancer-psychological-impact-family-caregivers

12. **U.S. National Library of Medicine.** *Physical and
Mental Health Effects of Family Caregiving*: 2008
Retrieved from https://www.ncbi.nlm.nih.gov/pmc/
articles/PMC2791523/

13. **American Psychological Association.** *Mental and
Physical Health Effects of Family Caregiving*: Retrieved
from http://www.apa.org/pi/about/publications/
caregivers/faq/health-effects.aspx

Made in the USA
Monee, IL
12 December 2020